Lunch Lessons

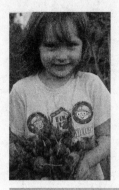 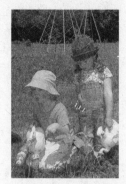 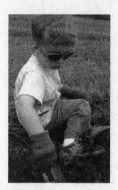

Lunch
Lessons

CHANGING THE WAY WE FEED OUR CHILDREN

ANN COOPER
AND
LISA M. HOLMES

 Collins

An Imprint of HarperCollins*Publishers*

HarperCollins books may be purchased for educational, business, or sales promotional use. For information please write to: Special Markets Department, HarperCollins Publishers, 10 East 53rd Street, New York, New York 10022.

First Collins paperback edition published 2007.

Designed by Ellen Cipriano

Library of Congress Cataloging-in-Publication Data is available.

ISBN: 978-0-06-078370-9 (pbk.)
ISBN-10: 0-06-078370-2 (pbk.)

07 08 09 10 11 ID/EOC 10 9 8 7 6 5 4 3

Dedication and Acknowledgments

Dedication:

Lunch Lessons is dedicated to all the lunch ladies and parents across this country who are working to provide children with wholesome, nutritious, delicious food. It is your passion and commitment that will rescue future generations from a lifetime of poor health. Keep fighting the good fight—it is one we simply cannot afford to lose.

Acknowledgments:

First and foremost we would like to thank Courtney Ross-Holst and the Ross School. It was Ross's vision for her extraordinary school that ultimately inspired us to take on the challenge of improving the National School Lunch Program and changing the way our children eat—forever. None of our work would have been possible without Ann's remarkable Ross School culinary team (specifically Beth Collins, Deena Chafetz, Coleen Donnelly, Chad Vanderslice, Evan Waters, and Robin Volinski) and the support of the school's faculty, staff, students, and parents. We thank each and every one of you for all you've done and continue to do. We are fortunate for the opportunity to share some of the school's recipes with the rest of the world in the pages of this book. We are grateful to Hailey London, the school's Registered Dietician who collaborated with us on Chapter I, Basic Childhood Nutrition, and helped Ann create the Healthy Kid's Meal Wheel.

Over the past several years we have met and worked with some extraordinary individuals who have inspired, educated, and generously given us their time, help, and guidance during the writing of *Lunch Lessons*. Working with Toni Liquori and Kate Adamick formerly of FoodChange, all of the EATWISE kids, and the Kellogg Foundation afforded us tremendous insight and gave us access to still more wonderful recipes for this book. Our gratitude, also, to Stephanie Sarka, an independent consultant working with the NYC Department of Education, Children First Initiative, for helping Toni reach her goals.

We are indebted to Alice Waters, Marsha Guerrerro, Chelsea Chapman, and Esther Cook with the Chez Panisse Foundation who also shared their favorite recipes and anecdotes as well as Zenobia Barlow and Janet Brown with the Center for Ecoliteracy for Rethinking School Lunch and sharing their vision with us. Michele Lawrence, superintendent of the Berkeley Unified School District, and Karen Trilevsky, founder of FullBloom Baking Company both played vital roles in shaping our thoughts for this project. FullBloom also generously donated recipes for the book. Many thanks, also, to all the others who gave their time for interviews and contributed their thoughts and ideas to the writing of this book.

A big thank-you also to Steve Murch at BigOven for his unparalleled help in getting our recipes moved and analyzed. All of our nutritional analyses were done using his fantastic software.

We are grateful for Herb Schaffner, our editor whose passion and dedication to this book have been unflagging, as well as to our agent, Lisa Ekus.

Finally we want to thank Lisa Macon, Michelle Wiesner, Alice Legarde, Nicole Findlay, and Jenny Hops who helped test recipes in their kitchens and at their dinner tables. Our heartfelt thanks also go out to Lisa's family, husband, John, and children, Ben and Kaia, who not only shared in the process of this work by tasting and critiquing recipes, but who also supported and brought into clearer focus the necessity of this work.

Contents

Foreword

Today we are in the throes of an obesity pandemic. Life expectancies are shorter. Thirty to forty percent of children born in the year 2000 will develop diabetes, and a great many of them will have other health problems resulting from obesity. As a surgeon who has dedicated my career to eradicating heart disease and other preventable diseases in adults, I cannot stress enough the importance of healthy diets for your children.

In order for us to combat the health impacts of the diseases related to obesity, we must change the way we feed children, as well as the way we educate them about food and how it relates to their health. The importance of this connection between diet and health cannot be overstressed.

Ann Cooper and Lisa M. Holmes are to be commended for taking a leadership role in the war to improve our children's health. As they raise their fists against the overuse of chemicals by agribusiness and the corporate infiltration of schools by fast food and processed-foods manufacturers, they present us with a wonderful guide, filled with in-depth research and delicious recipes, to changing our children's eating habits both at home and in school. Whether you are a parent, a teacher, a lunch lady, a school administrator, or just a caring individual, this book will change the way you think about school lunch.

Mehmet Oz
Professor and Vice Chair of Surgery
New York-Presbyterian/Columbia University

Authors' Note

In 1999 and 2000 we collaborated on *Bitter Harvest: A Chef's Perspective on the Hidden Danger in the Foods We Eat and What You Can Do About It* (Routledge 2000), a book whose purpose it was to raise public awareness not only of the pesticides, herbicides, genetically altered foods, and growth hormones that have infiltrated our food supply, but also to show how we can all work toward the long-term sustainability of the planet simply by changing the way we eat. How we purchase, prepare, and consume our foods matters deeply to our health as well as to the long-term health of the Earth. Our research for *Bitter Harvest* was wide and varied, but when we came across a piece of research that indicated that children born in the year 2000 would be the first in our country's history to die at a younger age than their parents, our focus was sharpened. We set about, in our own ways, to help kids make healthy changes in their lives. In this collaboration we come together as a mother and a school food advocate to bring you a collection of healthful recipes and helpful tips to forever change the way your children eat and live.

A man's palate can,
in time,
become accustomed
to anything.

—NAPOLEON BONAPARTE

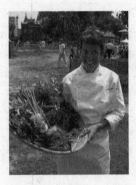

Introduction

Outside Mullen Hall, a Massachusetts public elementary school on Katherine Lee Bates Road just across from the Falmouth Public Library, there is, inevitably, a traffic jam just before nine o'clock each weekday morning. Caused in no small part by the crossing guard who works at a perplexing pace, the confusing beehive of activity seems endless. Children hurry out of minivans by the dozens, backpacks dragging the ground as they run toward the school's front door.

Since these children are still quite young, most aren't showing signs

Ann Cooper with harvest basket on the Washington Mall for the Smithsonian American Folk Life Festival *The Chez Panisse Foundation* of obesity yet, but if their eating habits don't change now they'll soon be on the wrong end of the statistics. Many already are. The percentage of obese children in America today has more than doubled since 1970. More than 35 percent of our nation's children are overweight, 25 percent are obese, and 14 percent have type 2 diabetes, a condition previously seen primarily in adults. Processed foods favored by schools and busy moms for their convenience not only contribute to obesity, they also contain additives and preservatives and are tainted with herbicide and pesticide residues that are believed to cause a variety of illnesses, including cancer. In fact, current research shows that 40 percent of all cancers are attributable to diet. Many hundreds of thousands of Americans die of diet-related illnesses each year. People in America today simply do not know how to eat properly, and they don't seem to have time to figure out how—so fast food, home meal replacements, and processed foods take the place of good, healthy cooking. There couldn't be a worse alternative.

Parents, pediatricians, and school administrators are increasingly concerned about children's health as it relates to diet. Most parents don't even know what constitutes good childhood nutrition and many feel they lack the time they would need to spend researching it. They rely, instead, on the USDA-approved National School Lunch Program (NSLP) to provide their children with nutritionally balanced, healthful meals. Trouble is, they're not. While most schools continue to try to meet better nutritional guidelines, they're still not measuring up, and many actually contribute to the crisis we've seen emerging over the last decade. Food is not respected; rather, it is something that must be made and consumed with increasing speed. In part, this is the result of the fact that there are more kids than ever in schools with smaller facilities, forcing several short lunch shifts. In many cases, decreasing budgets have also caused a decline in the quality of school meals.

For the most part, school lunch has deteriorated to institutional-style mayhem. Walk through the kitchen or lunchroom of almost any public or private school and "fast-food nation" will ring with striking clarity. USDA-approved portions of processed foods are haphazardly dished out by harried cafeteria workers to frenzied students hurrying to finish their food in time for ten minutes of recess. Nothing about the experience of being in a school cafeteria is calm—the din is deafening. Lunchrooms are vast open spaces filled with long tables flanked by dozens of chairs. There is no intimacy. No sense of calm. No respite from a morning of hard learning. Virtually all teachers hate lunchroom duty and view it as the most chaotic moment of their day—in fact, the New York City teachers' union recently won the right to stay outside the lunchroom. They now drop their students off at the cafeteria door on their way to find more restful lunchtime locations for themselves.

The noise and activity levels are not the only unpalatable aspects of lunchroom dining. A full 78 percent of the schools in America do not actually meet the USDA's nutritional guidelines, which is no surprise considering the fact that schools keep the cost of lunch between $1 and $1.50 per child. A parent in Colorado tells us that her child's school insists that nachos meet the dietary requirements for a main course. Horrified, she exclaimed, "It's not even real cheese!" The mother of an elementary student in Marstons Mills, Massachusetts, was appalled to learn that even apple slices aren't a nutritionally sound choice in her daughter's school—to her horror, they're topped with blue sugar sprinkles. Most kids do not even like the foods that are being served. A recent survey of school children in northern Minnesota revealed the food is so abysmal that not even old standby favorites like pizza and macaroni and cheese were given high marks. It's no wonder that kids are choosing fast foods, which are chemically engineered in many cases to be better tasting, over regular school lunch menu items. Kids today are bombarded with food advertising that is reinforced by the careful placement of fast-food chains in strip malls near schools and even on public school campuses. The big chains like McDonald's have been aggressively and specifically targeting children for decades. When Ray Kroc first started expanding the McDonald's chain, he would hop in a Cessna and fly around looking for prime real estate as close to schools as possible. Today they use satellite technology to locate the same type of properties. These companies are literally stalking our children. They've even found ways to get inside schools and be part of the public school lunch menus. A mother from Aurora, Colorado, told us that there is one Taco Bell and one Pizza Hut option available on every menu in her six-year-old son's lunchroom. She was told that the fast-food program originally started as a "safety measure" to keep the high school and middle school students on school grounds because in spite of the fact that they had a closed campus, kids were crossing busy streets to get to fast-food restaurants near their schools. She thought that "the fast-food thing just trickled down to the elementary program." Of course, the reality is that those schools were, and are, making money off million-dollar multiyear contracts with fast-food companies.

School lunch menus have undergone some changes in recent years and are marginally improved, but nearly all our schools continue to operate under the misguided notion that kids actually prefer to eat frozen, processed, fried, and sugary foods. Because most parents don't have time to spend in the kitchen the way the parents of generations past once did, the lunch lessons children are getting in school are the primary guideposts available to them. Poor in-school health and nutrition education is causing children, and by extension their families, to make bad food choices that are translating directly into big health problems. It is up to us, the consuming public, to not only get fast food out of our public schools, but to improve the quality of school lunches, from the nutritional content all the way to the atmosphere in our cafeterias. The money to fund school lunches comes directly out of our pockets and we need to set an example for our children that will keep them healthy now and help them to make better food choices in their adult lives. Everything we consume becomes part of us. Our food provides us with nourishment. It sustains us. It may also be our ultimate undoing. We literally are what we eat—good and bad. Changing the way we feed our children is not a luxury: It's an imperative. Concerned, informed, and involved parents and caregivers are the first line of defense.

The Path to Change

In spite of the ever increasing encroachment of fast food in the public school system, some schools and school districts have tried to change the way school meals are prepared, served, and eaten, but many have found the path toward change overwhelming. California's Berkeley High School made some recent strides toward creating an organic food court after the cafeteria there had been made unusable by the 1989 Loma Prieta earthquake. In 2001 the school reached out to local restaurateurs, such as the famed Alice Waters, who agreed to bring organic lunches to the school every day. Unfortunately, the program was poorly planned and inadequately executed. Only about 250 of the 3,000 students on campus ever ate in the food court. The vast majority of students did not even know the food court existed and those who did know about it quickly discovered that they could get the exact same lunches off-campus in bigger portions for less money. For several years the school abandoned its efforts, but in 2005 the Berkeley school district hired Ann Cooper. By the end of the 2006 school year, 90 percent of all the food served in the district was made from scratch. Fresh fruits and vegetables were served daily, and salad bars were installed in all the schools. Only a small percentage of the food is organic or local, but fresh, healthy foods are finally making their way onto children's plates.

The Ross School in East Hampton, New York, an alternative middle and high school with a curriculum based on cultural history, an emphasis on lifelong wellness, and a diverse community that ensures ever-expanding consciousness, did clean the slate, and now kids are clearing their plates—in more ways than one. Ann Cooper interviewed for the position of executive chef in 1999, at which point she met the founder, Courtney Ross, who shared her belief in the importance of eating healthful, nutritious, organic food. Ross wanted to implement a new lunch program at the Ross School that reflected her ideals. That simple exchange grew to eventually become R.O.S.S. (Regional Organic Seasonal Sustainable) food.

Over the many months the school's chefs collaborated in the kitchen before the new school café opened, Cooper watched the Ross School's food program change every person who worked there. Chad, the pastry chef, changed the way he fed his own children—every day. Deena, the school's executive sous-chef, stopped eating meat. People who had worked in professional kitchens all their adult lives gained a whole new respect for their profession and the food that they produced. From cooks to dishwashers and servers, not one person was left untouched, and that was only the beginning. As the program was put in place, teachers, students, farmers, the school's Executive Team, and even the laundry team, was changed. At Ross, food and nutrition are now a critical part of the school's underlying wellness program, and in the curriculum they are explicitly linked with exercise, health, and general well-being, both physical and mental. Ross has developed a successful, fiscally responsible, and utterly unique approach to mealtime that combines education, cooking lessons, and organic foods cooked to order by highly trained chefs. Now others are looking at R.O.S.S. food as a model for the future of school lunch programs around the country—even public schools.

Of course, it would be great if all schools would take the path Ross and other schools like Martin Luther King Junior Middle School (Edible Schoolyard) in Berkeley, California, have taken—then we'd all be able to rest easy knowing that our children were being served high quality, nutritious meals every day, but that day remains a long way off. Because we know how hard it can be to find something interesting and healthful to put in those lunch boxes every day, we've gathered together about 70 recipes from the Ross School (identified by R), Alice Waters's Chez Panisse Foundation (CPF), FullBloom Baking Company (FB), and the FoodChange (FC) that will help guide you in making better selections for your children. We've even included breakfast and snack recipes. First and foremost, however, it's important to have a clear understanding of basic childhood nutrition.

Lunch Lessons

EATING . . .
is more than deciding
what and when to eat.
FEEDING . . .
is more than choosing food
and getting it into a child.
EATING AND FEEDING . . .
reflect people's histories,
their relationships with
themselves and with others . . .

—ELLYN SATTER

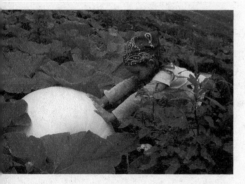

CHAPTER 1

Basic Childhood Nutrition

in collaboration with
Registered Dietician
Hailey London

When it comes to nutrition, children are not just miniature adults. Because they're growing, they have different dietary needs. When they start school, even preschool, it becomes more difficult to keep an eye on what they're eating. Since it's impossible for most parents to be with their school-age children at lunchtime during the week, the best you can do is send them to school with a healthy, well-balanced lunch. Start educating them early about what constitutes good nutrition so that when they're given the opportunity to make their own lunch choices they'll choose the best foods available to them.

Clementine with giant organic pumpkin *Sarah Pring*

Tips for Healthy Children

Eating habits are learned behaviors; they're not intuitive, so what your children learn to eat at home early in life sticks with them well into adulthood. Today we are disconnected from our food sources in a way that is unprecedented in human history. Fewer and fewer Americans cook meals from scratch because it's easier and faster to throw a frozen dinner in the oven or grab something from a fast-food restaurant on the way home from work. And the guerilla marketing foisted upon us by fast- and processed-food companies isn't helping. Most parents know that their kids are under continuous assault by corporate food advertising but feel frustrated by and even powerless against it. In reality, a few simple tools combined with a mantra of "variety, moderation, and balance" will provide you with all you need to ensure the long-term nutritional health of your child.

1. Be a good role model.

Most of the parents we know complain that their children refuse to eat healthfully and come to us in search of magic recipes that will put an end to mealtime madness. The real problem most often lies with the parents, not the kids. Most of us are so accustomed to eating out and buying prepared foods in the grocery store that we don't even know what good food is anymore. We can't line our cabinets with packaged cereals and sodas and expect our kids to eat like they were raised on a commune in rural Vermont. In order to be good role models we must educate ourselves first and then practice what we preach.

Doctors learn almost nothing about nutrition during their many years of education: In 2003 a nutrition course was required at only 40 percent of medical schools.

Breaking News: Pediatricians Suggest Changing the Way We Feed Babies

Years and years of early childhood feeding advice has just been turned on its head. Instead of rice cereal as baby's first food, doctors are now saying that, scientifically speaking, it may be better to offer babies 6 months and older just about everything the rest of the family eats (with a few exceptions, like honey, which is still recommended after the age of one). Even peanut butter before the first birthday isn't taboo. The reason for this sudden medical shift? For one thing, it's increasingly clear that eating habits are formed very early in life—perhaps even earlier than previously recognized, and keeping children on a diet of bland, simple foods may cause them to seek less variety in their diets as they get older, which can ultimately lead to problems with obesity.

Despite decades of consistent urgings by pediatricians across the country to keep things bland and simple, there's no hard scientific evidence to suggest that way is better than any other. In fact, science is actually suggesting that giving children heavily processed rice cereal as a first food may also be contributing to the obesity crisis because it is easily digested and raises blood sugar and insulin levels much more quickly than less processed foods would.

First-time parents are often afraid to stray from pediatricians' suggestions that early foods should be bland because they fear allergic reactions. The fact is that once a child reaches 6 months she can eat just about anything as long as foods are introduced one at a time to rule out potential allergies. A bit more caution is necessary if there is a family history of food allergies, but it's still largely safe to forge ahead with new foods earlier than most pediatricians have recommended in the past. It is well-documented that parents around the world have far less hesitation about giving their babies more zesty fare and not only does it work for them, obesity rates around the world are far lower than they are in the United States.

2. Take your kids shopping with you.

Unfortunately we don't all live near farms or farmers' markets, so it's not easy for us or our children to feel a connection with good, whole (unprocessed) foods. One way to help them learn is to make a point to take them grocery shopping with you. Of course it's probably easier to go alone when there's someone at home to watch them or they're at school, but it's important for them to see foods in their raw states so they can explore and ask questions. Take them when you're not in a hurry and spend a lot of time in the aisles that contain unprocessed foods—the produce, meat, and fish departments, for example. If your child appears to be interested in a certain type of fruit or vegetable, encourage him or her to explore that item; don't just assume that your child won't like it. Take it home and let him try it so he can make his own decisions. When Ben, Lisa's son, was a baby he liked to ride in the cart holding an avocado. Every time they went shopping he'd point at the avocados until Lisa gave him one. When he was three he asked if he could bring some mangos home. He was also intrigued by the spiky orange exterior of the unusual kiwano fruit (also known as the African Horned Melon). He carried it for the duration of their shopping trip and insisted it be cut the minute he got it home. Its green, seedy interior was a bit off-putting to him, but he tried it anyway. Exploring food this way gives Ben and his mom a chance to talk about how something is cooked and where it comes from. It also allows Ben to feel like he's making choices about what he eats.

3. Be flexible!

Remember, anything in moderation is okay. Of course, if you eat doughnuts in moderation, followed by potato chips in moderation and soda in moderation, it is no longer healthy. Having a cookie every day and balancing it with healthy foods is a better practice of moderation.

In 2002, a University of Michigan survey found that six of the sixteen hospitals ranked best in the country had fast-food franchises in them.

While we always want to make the healthiest choices for our children's bodies, a special treat once a week or even once a day won't do any damage. On the contrary, it will help make eating a more enjoyable experience and will help your child build a good relationship with food.

4. Make mealtime special.

There are all sorts of fun things we can do to make mealtime special. First and foremost, sit down and enjoy your food. Take time to savor flavors. Children should never eat while walking around. We understand that some young children have difficulty sitting for the entire meal. In those cases we recommend allowing the child to get up once or twice, while encouraging the child to sit—not stand—at the table when he or she comes back to eat. For children who are able to understand, explain to them that mealtimes are special family times and it is important to the family that everyone sit down to eat and talk together. Make a ritual out of dinner and give everyone a special task—maybe even let each child have one night a week to plan and help make dinner. Have the kids set the table. Cloth napkins and real glasses set a more formal tone and are better for the environment. Candles aren't just for adult dining—they can set a calming tone for the meal and will show kids that mealtime is special. Make a point not to allow mealtimes to degenerate into family argument time.

5. Don't be a short-order cook.

Ever find yourself making one meal for the adults in the house and another for the kids—or even one for each kid? Children take their time warming up to new things and if you keep giving them the old standbys they're not going to branch out and explore new foods. Be patient. Most research says that it takes an average of ten to twelve attempts before a child will try a new food, unless they are involved in cooking and gardening projects like Alice Waters's Edible Schoolyard (see page 65) or after school summer programs like The Magic Garden Club (see page 109). Learning about food and cooking in an active way helps breed a sense of culinary adventure. Make the same dinner for everyone in the family while making sure to put some foods on the plate that your children like—then add something new. If they don't touch it, don't worry about it, and definitely don't make an argument out of it. Try again the next week and again the following week. Eventually they'll surprise you by at least tasting that new food.

6. Don't buy into marketing for kids.

Kids don't need frozen chicken nuggets, French fries, macaroni and cheese, and pizza to keep them happy. And those kinds of foods certainly don't make for healthy children. Avoid processed foods at all costs and start talking to your children early in their lives about what constitutes a good diet and why it's important for them to avoid foods like the ones mentioned above. Even a three-year-old can grasp why sodas aren't good for you and why we don't eat foods with lots of fat every day at every meal. Highly processed foods are loaded with chemicals, synthetic fats, additives, artificial sweeteners, and food colorings. Ben bought an ice pop from the ice-cream man one summer afternoon at the beach with friends and when he got home his hand, leg, and face were blue—dark blue. It took several washings and a long bath to get the food coloring off his skin. Underneath the food-colored stains his skin was bright red and stayed red for several hours afterwards. Kids love brightly colored foods because advertising (kids see 10,000 food-related

Most of our food travels 1,500 miles before we eat it.

commercials a year!) trains them to believe that those foods are kid foods. Bright blue seems to be a favorite—everything from beverages to applesauce can be bought in a frightening shade of blue.

Faced with the child who thinks he might implode without that blue applesauce, hold your ground and look for an organic applesauce instead while explaining that both taste the same but one has things added to it that aren't healthful. If you have a particularly stubborn child do a blind taste test to prove your point. Parents should be working to remove food colorings, benzoate preservatives, and artificial sweeteners from their children's diets.

This is one battle parents and caregivers should be choosing to fight. More than 2.5 million children have been diagnosed with Attention Deficit Hyperactivity Disorder (ADHD) and an additional 15 percent of children have borderline hyperactivity or behavioral issues.[1] During our research we discovered nearly 100 studies validating the hypothesis that food dyes and additives are a factor in attention and behavior disorders and can increase the incidence of ADHD.[2] In one of those studies 73 percent of children placed on a diet free from chemical additives, dyes, and artificial sweeteners showed a reduction in hyperactivity and an increase in attention.[3]

Since television ads are the most prevalent medium and therefore influential, we recommend limiting television viewing early in life to PBS, which has fewer commercials than Nickelodeon and Noggin, or better yet, to videos with no commercials (be aware, however, that just like at the movie theater, many of today's releases do contain food advertising—use the fast forward button!). Use a digital video recorder to record special programs on television so you can edit out the commercials as they watch. It will, of course, be impossible to keep heavily processed foods

[1] "Attention-Deficit/Hyperactivity Disorder: A Public Health Perspective" (U.S. Department of Health and Human Services, Centers for Disease Control, 2002).

[2] J. L. Berdonces, "Attention Deficit and Infantile Hyperactivity," *Revista de enfermería* 24 (1; January 2001): 11–14. (Spanish).

[3] M. Boris and F. Mandel, "Foods and Additives are Common Causes of the Attention Deficit Hyperactive Disorder in Children," *Annals of Allergy* 72 (6; May 1994): 462–468.

Don't Super Size Your Kids

- Every day 1 in 4 Americans eats fast food.
- In the early 1970s Americans spent $3 billion on fast food. In 2004 we spent more than $110 billion.
- Of the two-thirds of 15-month-old American children who consume vegetables regularly, the top choice for most is French fries.
- Among children ages 6 to 19, 16 percent are considered overweight. That's more than 9 million American children.

Fast-Food Nutrition Facts

The average kid's meal at a fast-food restaurant might consist of a cheeseburger, small fries, and 16-ounce (small) soda. That meal may pack as many as 730 calories, nearly half of the recommended daily allowance for kids aged 4 to 6. A highly processed meal laced with additives, it also contains around 53 grams of fat (almost all the fat your child's body requires in a day), 3 tablespoons of sugar, and about half of the recommended daily allowance of sodium. Use the chart below to find the basic nutrition facts for your children's favorite fast-food items.

MENU ITEM	KCAL	TOTAL FAT (G)	SAT FAT (G)	KCAL FROM FAT (%)	SODIUM (MG)
Burger King Whopper	640	39	11	15	870
McDonald's Chicken McNuggets (9)	430	26	8	16	770
McDonald's Big Mac	560	31	10	16	1,070
McDonald's ¼ Pounder	420	21	8	17	820
w/cheese	530	30	13	22	1,290
McDonald's French Fries, large	450	22	9	17	290
McDonald's French Fries, small	220	11	2	45	150
McDonald's Chocolate Shake, 32 oz.	1,150	33	11	18	1,010
Burger King Double Whopper w/cheese	960	63	24	23	1,420
Jack in the Box Bacon Ultimate Cheeseburger	1,150	89	30	23	1,770
Burger King Cheeseburger	360	42	17	44	790
Hardee's Monster Burger	970	67	29	27	1,920

out of their diets forever because you won't be with them every minute of the day, but the longer you can limit exposure while instilling healthy eating habits, the more likely your children will be to make better choices for themselves when left to their own devices.

7. Don't use food as rewards, bribes, or punishments.

Okay, okay, we know, M&M's have a long history as the greatest bribe candy on Earth for potty training—even the most health-conscious mom will break down and try M&M's during that oh-so-critical stage of development. Don't give in! Stickers work just as well and you won't be setting a precedent for using food as a bribe or reward as your child gets older. Sure, it's okay to take the kids out for ice cream or frozen yogurt after a good (or even a bad) soccer game, just don't use it as an incentive for a good game. On the flip side, don't punish children for not eating certain foods—it will only foster a negative relationship between you and your children, not to mention your children and food.

8. Let kids help in the kitchen.

Encourage your children to help out in the kitchen. Even a two-year-old can help peel potatoes or carrots. For smaller children, invest in a stool, like The Learning Tower (www.heirloomwoodentoys.com), that allows your children to safely reach the kitchen counter so they can see what you're doing, or if you have room, set up a workstation at your child's height so he can participate without having to stand on tiptoes. Taller children may only need a small wooden stepstool to reach a comfortable height. If a child is interested in doing more in the kitchen, don't automatically assume that she can't or that the task will be too

As much as 70 percent of all antibiotics consumed in this country are utilized in animal husbandry.

Ten Things Parents Can Do to Help Prevent Eating Disorders

From the National Eating Disorders Association, Michael P. Levine, PhD, and Margo D. Maine, PhD, 2003

1. Accept your body and your child's body at any weight and help them to understand (a) the genetic basis for the natural diversity of human body shapes and sizes and (b) the nature and ugliness of prejudice.

- Make an effort to maintain positive attitudes and healthy behaviors. Children learn from the things you say and do! It's about being healthy, not looking a certain way!

2. Examine closely your dreams and goals for your children and other loved ones. Are you overemphasizing beauty and body shape, particularly for girls?

- Avoid conveying an attitude which says in effect, "I will like you more if you lose weight, don't eat so much, look more like the slender models in ads, fit into smaller clothes, etc."
- Decide what you can do and what you can stop doing to reduce the teasing, criticism, blaming, staring, etc. that reinforce the idea that larger or fatter is "bad" and smaller or thinner is "good."

3. Learn about and discuss with your sons and daughters (a) the dangers of trying to alter one's body shape through dieting, (b) the value of moderate exercise for health, and (c) the importance of eating a variety of foods in well-balanced meals consumed at least three times a day.

- Avoid categorizing and labeling foods (e.g., good/bad or safe/ dangerous). All foods can be eaten in moderation.
- Be a good role model in regard to sensible eating, exercise, and self- acceptance.

4. Make a commitment not to avoid activities (such as swimming, sunbathing, dancing, etc.) simply because they call attention to your weight and shape. Refuse to wear clothes that are uncomfortable or that you don't like but wear simply because they divert attention from your weight or shape.

5. Make a commitment to exercise for the joy of feeling your body move and grow stronger, not to purge fat from your body or to compensate for calories, power, excitement, popularity, or perfection.

6. Talk candidly to your children about any pressures they may feel to diet or look good. Help children to understand the negative physical, social, and emotional consequences of dieting.

7. Help children appreciate and resist the ways in which television, magazines, and other media distort the true diversity of human body types and imply that a slender body means power, excitement, popularity, or perfection.

8. Trust your children's appetites. Do not limit their caloric intake unless a physician requests that you do this because of a medical problem. Avoid rewarding or punishing children with food. This adds to the emotional meaning that food can assume.

9. Encourage your children to be active and to enjoy what their bodies can do and feel like.

10. Do whatever you can to promote the self-esteem and self-respect of all of your children in intellectual, athletic, and social endeavors. Give boys and girls the same opportunities and encouragement. Be careful not to suggest that females are less important than males, e.g., by exempting males from housework or child care. A well-rounded sense of self and solid self-esteem are perhaps the best antidotes to dieting and disordered eating.

dangerous. Know your child's limits and help him achieve success by providing support and encouragement in a safe setting. Kids love eating food they create. Involve your child in the cooking or snack preparation and they will be more likely to eat new foods, including fruits and vegetables.

75 percent of the antibiotics in this country have become ineffective against many diseases.

9. *Love and accept your child no matter what!*

Love and accept your child at any weight, size, or shape. During childhood, growth is unpredictable at best. It comes in spurts and a once-skinny child can suddenly plump up while his height catches up with his weight. There's a lot of pressure in our society to be thin and you might be tempted to put your child on a diet during a growth spurt, but that won't be helpful and may even cause emotional and physical damage. Instead, help your child maintain his weight until his height catches up. The best way to do that is to teach good healthy eating habits.

10. *Make sure your child eats breakfast.*

It's the most important meal of the day, and it should ideally be the largest meal of the day to get your child off on the right foot. After ten to twelve hours with no food it's important to refuel the engines. If they don't eat in the morning they'll be tired and unable to concentrate in school before lunch. It's essential that children jumpstart their metabolism in the morning so their bodies don't enter starvation mode, which might later cause them to experience difficulty maintaining a healthy body weight.

Some children need to practice eating breakfast. We recommend starting small and working to a bigger meal if you're having trouble getting your child to eat breakfast. For most children, breakfast should be around 500 calories and should be nutritionally balanced. Starting kids off with sugar first thing in morning is not ideal. This gives a quick burst of energy and then leaves your child drained. Breakfast should always include a source of protein, some healthy fats, carbohydrates (whole grains are best), and vitamins and minerals. A great breakfast

E. coli is resistant to almost all antibiotics.

for a family with time in the morning would be two eggs, whole-wheat toast, fruit, or hot wholegrain cereal or wholegrain low-fat granola and 100 percent fruit juice. A family with less time might choose a hard-boiled egg to go with a slice or two of wholegrain toast, or a peanut butter and jelly sandwich on whole-wheat bread.

Many schools now offer free breakfast universally to children. If your child does not have time to eat breakfast at home, make sure he eats at school.

11. Encourage your children to move their bodies.

A good diet is only part of the equation. In order to stay healthy our bodies need exercise. Studies have shown that vigorous exercise boosts the immune system and increases our ability to concentrate. Help your children find physical activities they enjoy and encourage them to get outside to play as often as possible.

Identifying age-appropriate activities will make exercise more fun. Children between the ages of 2 and 5 enjoy simple activities—running, jumping, kicking a ball, riding a tricycle (a bicycle as they get closer to age 5), and even using their imagination to trot and gallop like a horse or hop like a kangaroo. Backyard play is best for this age group, while for kids between age 5 and 8 organized, noncompetitive sports can be extremely rewarding. Roller-skating and ice-skating can be introduced at this age. Encourage your 5- to 8-year-old to explore a wide variety of sports and physical activities to allow her to begin to discover her likes and dislikes. Children ages 9 and up enjoy competitive team sports, but puberty can make many teens feel self-conscious and awkward, especially around their peers. Help them find activities, like yoga, strength training, jogging, and aerobic dancing, that can be done as part of a group or solo. Every once in a while a family hike makes a great change of pace for all ages.

As with eating, a parent's good example can make the difference for a child. Make sure exercise is a part of your daily routine as well.

12. *Remember that you are the boss.*

Adults need to set the boundaries for kids because left to their own de-vices they may choose salty and sugary processed foods over fresh, healthier choices. Children actually do much better when they know that they have boundaries and limits. Listen to your child, but set clear limits and guide them toward the healthier option.

Chef Ann's Guide to Healthy Eating

Figuring out how to put together a balanced, appropriate-sized meal can be a challenge in today's world, especially because food isn't what it used to be. And because of that we're not exactly well-equipped to make the right choices. Bagels and muffins are good examples of how once-innocuous foods have turned into high-calorie, high-fat mon-strosities. Years ago the average muffin contained about 140 calories. Today they pack anywhere from 350 to 600 calories. Most restaurant meals, especially at mid-priced family-style establishments, are much too large for the average adult. For the average child they're completely off the map.

Advertising, a sort of corporate guerilla warfare, reinforces the new norms and sets nutritional land mines for all of us. If it's becoming dif-ficult for adults to understand what constitutes a properly portioned, healthful meal for themselves, it's no wonder that most parents feel completely lost when it comes to proper childhood nutrition. Add to that the fact that children watch an average of 10,000 food-related commercials a year, a large portion of which are for high-calorie, low-nutrient foods, forcing parents into an instant uphill battle to entice their children to eat good, wholesome foods.

Children of different ages and activity levels have different nutri-tional requirements. The following guide to healthy eating will help you figure out what is appropriate for your children.

Chef Ann's Healthy Kid's Meal Wheel: A Guide for Making Healthy Food Choices Daily

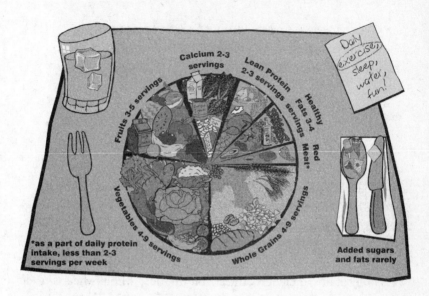

Total Daily Calorie Needs

The recommended number of food group servings depends on your calorie needs:

650 calories is about right for children 0 to 6 months
850 calories is about right for children 6 months to 1 year
1300 calories is about right for children 1 to 3 years
1600 calories is about right for children 4 to 6 years
2200 calories is about right for most children over 6 and teen girls
2800 calories is about right for teen boys

In the past four years, more than 40 varieties of crops have been genetically engineered, including more than 50 percent of our soybeans and 25 percent of our corn—these two crops alone impact more than *two-thirds* of the foods in grocery stores today.

Whole Grains:

- Children ages 6 to 9 should aim for 4 to 7 servings daily
- Children ages 10 to 14 should aim for 5 to 8 servings daily
- Teens ages 14 to 18 should aim for 6 to 9 servings daily

A serving is:

1 small slice of bread or ½ bagel the size of a hockey puck (If you buy a regular bagel from a bagel store, ½ bagel is usually equivalent to two servings of grains)
½ cup cooked rice equals what fits inside a cupcake wrapper
½ cup pasta
1 cup of whole grains

Whole grains include oatmeal, brown rice, whole-wheat bread/tortillas/pitas, quinoa, millet, bulgur, buckwheat, and barley, whole-grain cereals (look for fiber higher than 2 grams), whole-wheat pasta and other wholegrain breads. Refined grains, such as white flour, white pasta, and white rice should be limited to 3 to 4 times a week.

Vegetables:

- 4 to 9 servings daily (1 cup raw or ½ cup of cooked vegetables is one serving)

The more the better, just as long as smaller kids save room for protein and fats (essential to brain development) as well. When it comes to vegetables, go for a variety of colors like green, orange, red, purple blue, yellow, and white, to ensure that children are getting all needed vitamins and minerals and phytochemicals. Fresh and in season is always best. Organic is ideal, but the first and most important step is

Low-Carb/No Carb?

Although many adults feel that carbohydrates don't work well for them if they're trying to maintain their weight, children still have a great need for carbohydrates. A child's body should not be subjected to the strain that a carbohydrate-free diet puts on the body. Children need carbohydrates for energy, but should avoid those that are sugary or break down into sugar quickly. White bread, white pasta, and white rice convert very quickly to sugar, leaving your child drained after the initial burst of energy. Sugars and high-fructose corn syrup wreak havoc on growing children's bodies, depleting their immune systems, adding unnecessary calories, and impairing their focus.

Start children on wholegrain, fiber-rich carbohydrates while they're young so they don't grow accustomed to white bread, pasta, and white rice. Wholegrain products such as whole-wheat bread, oatmeal, brown rice, bulgur, quinoa, and cereal grains break down more slowly in the body, keeping a kid's energy level on an even keel. They also provide essential nutrients and fiber that kids need for growth and removal of toxins from the body.

to eat those veggies in any form. Some kids need to see or try a vegetable ten to twelve times before they accept it, so don't give up. Watch out for the starchy vegetables. While potatoes and corn have some nutrients, they have much less than most vegetables and are more like carbohydrates nutritionally. If potatoes or corn is served, a grain is not needed. Leave the skin on potatoes and carrots for extra nutrients.

- Add vegetables to pureed soups
- Keep a snack of raw vegetables and dip on hand in the refrigerator

Since WWII, pesticide use has risen tenfold and crop loss due to pests has doubled.

- Add vegetables to pizza
- Experiment with foods from other cultures, using a wide variety of vegetables. Sometimes a kid who won't touch a carrot or a piece of broccoli will happily eat it if it's cooked a different way

Fruits:

- 3 to 5 servings daily

The serving size for fresh fruit is about the size of a tennis ball, if whole. Most apples are a bit over a serving and half a banana is usually equivalent to one full fruit serving. For cut fruit, the serving size is ½ cup. For juice, ½ cup is a good size—take note that this is only 4 ounces and many "juice" glasses are 6, 8, or even 10 ounces. Make sure juice is 100 percent juice; otherwise it most likely has a high proportion of sugar and you might as well just be giving your kids soda.

Fresh is better than canned and syruped. Some snacks like fruit chews are heavy on sugar and high-fructose corn syrup. Fruit leathers from the health food store or organic section of the grocery store would be a good alternative to processed fruit snacks. If your child won't eat whole fruit, experiment with a wide variety of juices. Apple and orange juices are good, but mix it up a little. Some kids will gladly drink blueberry, peach, pear, mango, and even carrot juice. School-age children should try to eat a minimum of 3 or 4 servings of fruits daily. As with vegetables, aim for variety. While fruit is a healthy choice, it still can not be eaten without limit the way vegetables can because it contains significant calories and sugars.

U.S. agriculture uses 1.2 billion pounds of pesticides each year—roughly 5 pounds for every American.

Tips for adding more fruit to your child's diet:

- Always have some fresh fruit available in the kitchen
- Try fresh fruit salad for dessert
- Fruit Smoothies (page 148) are another good snack or an accompaniment to a meal
- Make some Chocolate–Peanut Butter Bananas (page 152) and keep them in the freezer for an on-the-go snack

Calcium:

- 2 to 6 servings daily
- Preschool-age children need 500 to 800 mg of calcium daily (2 to 3 servings)
- School-age children need about 800 mg daily (3 servings)
- Adolescents need about 1200 to 1500 mg of calcium daily (5 to 6 servings), which is a huge increase from preadolescence

You may be accustomed to seeing the USDA's dairy group, but we've replaced it with a calcium group because while calcium is the most important component of dairy, it is possible to get it, minus the fat, in other ways. Many plant sources contain calcium that is more readily absorbed by the body than the calcium found in dairy. Some examples include nuts, broccoli, dark leafy greens (add some lemon to help free up the calcium), tofu, soy milk, sardines, beans, sunflower seeds, and molasses. When getting calcium from dairy, the best source is organic yogurt, and the next best is low-fat or skim organic milk and other low-fat or nonfat organic dairy products. (Pediatricians recommend giving children under age 2 whole milk and then switching to skim after the second birthday.) Conventionally farmed dairy carries toxins and a variety of farming residues. If milk is the only organic food in your house you are still doing your family a great service, so if you prefer to eat dairy, please choose organic.

rBGH

Cattle normally produce hormones that regulate growth and milk production naturally. Relatively recently, however, Monsanto bio-engineered a replica hormone called Recombinant Bovine Growth Hormone (rBGH) or Bovine Somatotrophin (rBST), that can be administered to cows by dairy farmers to enhance, or increase, milk output. It appeared on the market in 1994 and has been used by a large segment of commercial U.S. diary operators since its approval by the FDA, an organization ostensibly dedicated to the protection of U.S. citizens. The FDA and Monsanto say that rBGH milk and rBGH-free milk are the same, but the truth is that the two are quite different. Saturated fatty acids are higher in rBGH milk as are levels of antibiotics because rBGH increases the cows' susceptibility to chronic mastitis and, as a result, antibiotic use in rBGH cows is higher. More antibiotics in milk means greater risk of allergic reactions in people as well as increased resistance. Mastitis produces pus, which also finds its way into the milk. Possibly the most serious problem with rBGH milk is that it contains high –levels of naturally occurring Insulin-like Growth Factor 1 (IGF-1), which regulates cell growth in humans, especially infants and children. Eli Lilly revealed that IGF-1 blood levels of cows treated with rBGH are up to ten times higher than in cows not given the hormone. IGF-1 is not broken down by pasteurization or digestion and is widely regarded as a major cause of cancer—particularly breast and colon cancer.

A 1998 study, based on 300 healthy nurses, showed that elevated IGF-1 blood levels are strongly associated with up to a sevenfold increased risk of developing premenopausal breast cancer. This is the highest known risk, approximating to that of a strong family history. More recent studies have also shown strong associations between increased IGF-1 blood levels and prostate cancer.

Of related concern is evidence that elevated IGF-1 levels inhibit the body's normal ability to protect itself from microscopic cancers by the natural process of programmed cell destruction, known as "apoptosis." This promotes the growth and invasiveness of early cancers, and also decreases their responsiveness to chemotherapy."*

As far back as 1999 a European Commission report (http://europa.eu.int/comm/food/fs/sc/scv/out19_en.html#_Toc446393146) stated that one of the best ways to prevent cancer would be to simply avoid dairy products tainted with rBGH. We wholeheartedly agree.

*Sources: Eng-Hen Ng et al., "Altered Serum Levels of Insulin-like Growth-Factor Binding Proteins in Breast Cancer Patients," *Annals of Surgical Oncology* 5 (2; March 1998): 194–201 and A. Wolk et al., "Insulin-like Growth Factor 1 and Prostate Cancer Risk: A Population-based, Case-control Study," *Journal of the National Cancer Institute* 90 (1998): 991–915.

The serving size of calcium-rich foods varies based on the amount of calcium in the food. For a serving of calcium, try:

- 1 cup of cooked beans: soy, white, navy, black, french, refried, winged, and great Northern have the most calcium
- $\frac{1}{2}$ cup almonds
- $\frac{1}{2}$ cup dried figs
- 3 ounces canned salmon
- 6 canned sardines
- 1 cup amaranth (ancient grain)
- $\frac{1}{2}$ cup dark leafy green vegetables, cooked (collards, kale, spinach, escarole, beet greens, etc.)
- $\frac{1}{2}$ cup tofu
- 1 cup low-fat milk or soy milk
- 1 cup low-fat yogurt
- $1\frac{1}{2}$ ounces low-fat cheese

Lean Protein:

- 2 to 3 servings daily (A serving is 2 to 3 ounces of meat, $\frac{1}{2}$ cup of cooked beans, $\frac{1}{3}$ cup of nuts, or one egg)

Mercury in Fish

Lately there's been a great deal reported in the media about mercury in fish. Most recently an article was published in the *Wall Street Journal*[1] that spotlighted the case of a fifth grader who had a penchant for canned tuna. At the height of his tuna consumption he was eating 3 to 6 ounces of the fish per day. During the school year the boy began to lose focus, couldn't do simple math, and became disinterested in school in general. His parents noticed that his sports abilities were waning as well. Worried, they took him to see a neurologist who ordered blood work. The results were shocking. The boy had mercury levels in his blood that were nearly double what the EPA considers safe.

The EPA's methylmercury guideline is a recommended limit on mercury consumption based on body weight, also known as a "reference dose." EPA's methylmercury reference dose is .1 micrograms/kg body weight per day.

How much canned tuna can a 40-pound child safely ingest in one week?

- Convert 40 pounds to kilograms: $40 \times .45 = 18$ kilograms
- 18 kilograms $\times$ .1 micrograms per kilogram per day = 1.8 mcg per kg per day
- EPA LEVEL CONSIDERED SAFE = 1.8 micrograms per day $\times$ 7 days = 12.6 micrograms per week.)

The average 6-ounce can of white albacore tuna contains approximately 58 micrograms of mercury (some estimates are significantly higher).

Even Half a Can of Tuna is *More Than Four and a Half Times* What is Considered Safe by the EPA for a 40-Pound Child.

It's frightening, we know, but unpolluted fish are good for you and your children. They're high in omega-3s, which are known to maintain and improve cardiovascular health. Don't cut fish out of your child's diet, but make a point to know which fish are clean using the conversion factor above rather than accepting so called "safe" serving sizes, and avoid canned tuna altogether.

Oceans Alive is a great source for information about the safety of a wide variety of food fish. They also have a clear, simple chart that indicates the number of

times a certain type of fish can be safely eaten per month (www.oceansalive
.org/eat.cfm?subnav=shouldiworry).

Another group, the Blue Ocean Institute (blueocean.org/seafood) currently recommends walleye pollock and Alaska salmon as the best environmental choices.

[1]Peter Waldman, "Fish Line Mercury and Tuna: U.S. Advice Leaves Lots of Questions Balancing
Interests, Agencies Issue Guidance at Odds With EPA Risk Assessment: A Schoolboy's Sudden
Setback," *The Wall Street Journal*, August 1, 2005, p. A1.

A growing body needs protein every day. Healthy protein sources
include nuts, beans, tofu, fish (wild is most often better than farm-
raised), eggs, chicken, turkey, lean pork, and lamb. Although fish is a
great source of protein, canned tuna should be consumed very infrequently (see box above) due to mercury. Chunk light tuna has a lower
concentration of mercury than chunk white tuna. Cheese has some
protein, but it is high in saturated fat. Only allow your children to eat
high-saturated-fat proteins like cheese, bacon, sausage, hot dogs, and
salami once in a while. Children, like adults, need about 3 servings of
protein a day. Many children actually get too much protein because
the majority of adults are not aware of how small a portion of protein
truly is.

Healthy Fats:

• 3 to 4 servings daily

Fats from plant sources are very important to the growth and development of children's bodies. Limit animal fats, which contain saturated
fat and cholesterol. Eliminate trans-fatty acids that come from food

---

The CDC has stated that obesity is overtaking cigarette smoking as the number one cause of preventable death in America.

---

that is hydrogenated by checking labels and avoiding food with the word *hydrogenated* in the ingredients.

Healthy fats include oils such as olive, safflower, sesame, flax, and canola. A serving of these oils is 1 teaspoon. Note: Flax oil should not be heated or used for cooking.

A serving of nuts like almonds, walnuts, and peanuts for healthy fat is a handful, or a bit less than ½ cup; 1 tablespoon peanut, almond, or cashew butter also constitutes one serving.

Legumes, such as peas, beans, lentils, chick peas (garbanzos), soy beans, tofu, and soy products also contain healthy fats. One serving is 1 cup cooked.

Note: If consuming beans and nuts for healthy fats, you will be getting a serving of calcium with these foods, as well.

Red Meat:

- 2 to 3 servings per week

Red meat was separated out from the proteins, not to encourage you to eat it, but to reinforce that it should be consumed very infrequently. In this category would also be bacon, ham, sausage, salami, bologna, and hot dogs (unless 100 percent turkey, or vegetarian, and low-fat). These meats contain a large proportion of saturated fat and should be eaten in moderation for heart health. When choosing red meat, look for natural or organic beef.

The early onset of puberty and menopause in women and lowered semen counts in men have been traced in part to food additives and poor diet.

Added Sugars and Fats:

• To be eaten rarely

Although kids may think sugar is their best friend, it's more like their worst enemy. Much of today's obesity crisis stems from lack of exercise and heavy eating of foods with minimal nutritional value. Sugary foods are a big part of that problem. Empty calories from soda, candy, snacks, and cereals add up, causing weight problems and mood swings in children. High-fructose corn syrup, found in many foods, is not healthy, especially for children. Adding a soda a day to a child's diet has been shown to increase his weight by as much as 20 to 30 pounds each year. It is believed that soda consumption is a major contributor to today's obesity epidemic. What about artificially sweetened sodas? Diet sodas aren't good for kids either because products like Nutrasweet and Splenda have not been tested thoroughly enough. Preliminary results have shown that these unnatural sugars are not great for kids. Additionally, kids should never be given soda with caffeine, as it is harmful to a growing body. Limit soda, candy, and sugary snacks, and balance them with healthy foods.

Foods with high quantities of added sugars, such as candy, soda, cakes, pies, and cookies, should be limited to treats. For very active kids, a daily treat in moderation can be part of a healthy diet. Kids who are not as physically active should really limit high-sugar foods and beverages to a few times per week.

Growing bodies need healthy fats. Added fats, especially hydrogenated fats, should be reduced significantly. We recommend eliminating trans fats entirely (see box p. 26). Fats found in many fried foods, chips, fatty meats, and baked goods are not healthful. Choose fats from vegetable oils (not hydrogenated and not deep fried), nuts, fish, soy, avocado, olives, and lean chicken, turkey, and beef. Fried foods and heavy, fatty foods (cream sauces, very cheesy foods (like nachos), hot dogs, salami, bologna, and bacon, for example) should be limited to only a few times a week. Children need an ample amount of fat in their

Just Say No to Trans-Fatty Acids

In 2003, Stephen Joseph, a San Francisco public interest attorney, filed suit against Nabisco, claiming that the filling in Oreo cookies was so dangerous it shouldn't be marketed and sold to children who don't know what constitutes good nutrition. Medical research was showing that trans-fatty acids were far more dangerous than saturated fats, and consumers were largely unaware that they were being used so extensively in processed-food products. After the media frenzy that ensued, Joseph's lawsuit was no longer viable so he dropped it, but his mission had been accomplished. People everywhere were talking about killer trans fats.

Is it really all that dramatic? Can trans-fatty acids, also known as hydrogenated (or partially hydrogenated) oils, really kill you?

Well, the National Academy of Science's Institute of Medicine has said that trans fats shouldn't be eaten at all, and a study released by the American Heart Association "in 2002 showed that food cooked with trans fat clogs arteries quicker than food cooked in animal-based saturated fat."[1]

Trans fats act like saturated fats in the body, raising the levels of LDL, or "bad" cholesterol. Both saturated and trans fats "scrub" away HDL, or the "good" cholesterol that normally works to keep arteries clean. Since the ill effects of trans fats occur with greater speed than that of the average saturated fat, there is likely something else going on with these chemically altered fats. Kim Severson, author of *The Trans Fat Solution* reports that

> trans fat has what researchers are beginning to agree is a more insidious function in the body: It actually reprograms how cells work, causing lifelong damage that can lead to diabetes, stroke, and possibly cancer. Unlike saturated fats from animals, trans fats aren't easily broken down in the body. The molecular structure of trans fat is so different, so unnatural, that the body has no way to know exactly how to process it. That's why some doctors, in particular the top nutrition and heart experts at Harvard University, believe trans fat is worse than saturated fat.[2]

Trans-fatty acids are, in fact, everywhere in the American diet. This is nothing new, however. They've been a part of the American diet since the early 1900s when William Normann discovered the process of hydrogenating oils, making them easier to store and more shelf-stable than liquid fats. The difference is that today, because we eat so much fast food and heavily processed food, we consume in excess of 2,000 percent more trans fats than our ancestors did. Margarine and vegetable shortenings top the list of trans-fatty offenders, and processed foods are loaded with them. They add creaminess, crispness, and moisture to a wide variety of foods while prolonging shelf life and keeping manufacturing costs low. Fast-food restaurants love trans fats because they can take the abuse of repeated high temperatures in deep fat fryers.

Our kids, as usual, are the ultimate guinea pigs because they are major consumers of processed and fast foods. Because today's children eat about 40 percent of their meals in fast-food restaurants, they're consuming huge quantities of trans fats. And lest you think newborn babies are safe, research has shown that even before infants begin eating table foods they're ingesting them. Mary G. Enig, PhD, is a nutritionist who is widely recognized for her research on fats and oils, and a leading expert on trans fats. Enig says, "Canadian researchers found that infants consume fatty acids through their mother's milk. They followed this group of children up to 14 months and found that the higher the level of trans fats in the mother's diet, the less visual acuity the children had."[3]

The best thing to do is avoid trans fats whenever possible, and the easiest way to do that is to simply not buy processed foods. Use raw products and substitute butter for vegetable shortening and margarine in recipes. If you have to buy processed foods, be sure to read labels (the FDA is just now, in 2006, requiring manufacturers to list trans fats in their ingredients lists) and try not to buy anything that lists hydrogenated or partially hydrogenated oils.

Research shows that 40 percent of all cancer is diet-related.

diets for good growth and development. Roughly 30 percent of their daily calories should be from fat, and of the 30 percent, one-third or less should be from saturated fat.

Dietary Fats			
TYPE OF FAT	MAIN SOURCE	STATE AT ROOM TEMPERATURE	EFFECT ON CHOLESTEROL LEVELS
Monounsaturated	Olives; olive oil, canola oil, peanut oil; cashews, almonds, peanuts, and most other nuts; avocados	Liquid	Lowers LDL; raises HDL
Polyunsaturated	Corn, soybean, safflower, and cottonseed oils; fish	Liquid	Lowers LDL; raises HDL
Saturated	Whole milk, butter, cheese, and ice cream; red meat; chocolate; coconuts; coconut milk, and coconut oil	Solid	Raises both LDL and HDL
Trans	Most margarines; vegetable shortening; partially hydrogenated vegetable oil; deep-fried chips; many fast foods; most commercial baked goods	Solid or semisolid	Raises LDL

1. Kim Severson and Cindy Burke, *The Trans Fat Solution* (Berkeley: Ten Speed Press, 2003), 8.
2. Ibid.
3. Kelly Burgess, "Uh-oh, Oreos: The Trans Fats Debate" recipestoday.com/resources/articles/transfats.htm

Table source: www.hsph.harvard.edu/nutritionsource/fats.html

Water:

Hydration is vital to total body and brain health for growing kids. Every function of the human body requires water. Eight glasses a day should be the goal for water-drinking skeptics and a minimum for experienced water drinkers. Give your young children water, rather than juice or soda, when they're thirsty and they'll be more likely to choose water when they're older. Sugary drinks end up using more water than they provide, so go for water or seltzer. If your kids absolutely have to have flavored beverages, pour them a glass of seltzer and add a splash of fruit juice. Kids often drink more water if they are able to carry a water bottle at school.

Chef Ann's Healthy Kids Nutrition Report Card

It's not easy to keep a mental tally of what your kids are eating every day (especially if you have more than one child!), so we suggest using Chef Ann's Healthy Kids Nutrition Report Card to keep track. At the end of each day make an evaluation—did your child get most (Good) or all (Better) of the recommended servings in each category? If so, were they organic and local (Best)? Sit down with your kids at the end of the day and go over the report card with them—it's a great opportunity for a daily reminder of the importance of healthy eating.

Chef Ann's Healthy Kids Nutrition Report Card

NAME

STUDENTS ages 6 to 18*

EVALUATED BY www.lunchlessons.org

Official Grading Scale below FOOD CHOICES	Goals	Good	Better	Best
Vegetables	4-9 servings			
Fruits	3-5 servings			
Whole Grains	4-9 servings			
Lean Protein	2-3 servings			
Healthy Fats	3-4 servings			
Calcium	2-3 servings			
Red Meat	less than 2-3 servings per week			
Added sugars and fats	rarely			

Grading Scale:
Good = Met most requirements
Better = Met all requirements
Best = Met all requirements with local and organic ingredients

* younger ages = less servings

Daily Checklist:
exercise
sleep
water
safety
fun

Chef Ann's Healthy Kids Nutrition Report Card was developed by Chef Ann Cooper, in collaboration with Hailey London, R.D.

Exercise and recreation . . .
are as necessary as reading.
I will rather say more
necessary because health is
worth more than learning.

— THOMAS JEFFERSON

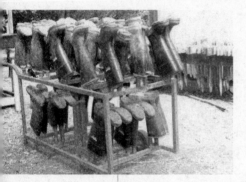

CHAPTER 2

Putting the Lesson in Lunch

Learning about childhood nutrition and changing the way you cook at home are the first steps toward change, but there is so much more work to be done if we're going to save this generation of children from the plague of obesity and poor nutrition. For us it means writing, giving speeches, and getting into schools to educate students, their parents, and school lunch providers and administrators. For you, it means getting out there and getting involved, and in this chapter we hope to inspire you with examples of programs and initiatives that work. While there is no one right answer to changing the way our children eat, it is

Boots for the Edible Schoolyard students *The Chez Panisse Foundation* important that all of you feel empowered to take back the responsibility of providing the children in your home and wider community with high-quality whole foods and the knowledge and power to make better choices in the future.

Why Do This?

It may seem utterly overwhelming to take on something as large as the National School Lunch Program (NSLP), and it would no doubt be infinitely easier just to use the recipes in this book and cook more healthfully for your own children than it would be to take on the larger system. But for us, there are two major reasons to fight this fight. First, we have a moral obligation. If we don't start working to get our nation's children on a path to better health, their life expectancy will decrease, health insurance premiums will further skyrocket, and the sustainability of our food supply will be at great risk. The second reason is that kids learn habits, both good and bad, around their peers. Peer influence can be stronger than parental influence—if all the cool kids eat fast food, fast food will be the food of choice no matter what Mom and Dad are cooking at home. If we're going to make the necessary changes, our battles must be taken to the front lines. It's not about changing the entire National School Lunch Program at once, it's about changing one school and one district at a time, just as the early proponents of the NSLP did.

A Brief History of School Lunch

Most people assume that the school lunch program is a modern American initiative. Not so. The very first school lunch program was started in Europe in the 1700s after teachers noticed that poor, malnourished children were having more difficulty concentrating than their well-fed classmates. Even more than three centuries ago the ill effects of poor nutrition on health and education were so abundantly clear that they could not be ignored. The earliest programs were funded through the efforts of private charities with the humble goal of providing the most nutritious meals at the lowest possible cost—hallmarks that remain part of school lunch programs around the world today. When philanthropies could no longer support the needs of their communities, local and national governments stepped in to help. Parents were relieved to know that not only were their children being fed, but that school attendance was soaring. At the same time, governments were able to almost guarantee themselves a larger number of healthier men to enlist in the armed services. Right from the beginning the primary motivating factors behind school food programs were both charitable and political. The first American school food programs, which started decades later, were no exception to this rule.

Major cities were among the first to put school food programs in place. Ellen H. S. Richards, home economics pioneer and the first woman admitted to the Massachusetts Institute of Technology (MIT), helped open the New England Kitchen in 1890. Its purpose was to provide nutritious yet inexpensive food to working-class families in Boston while teaching them the principles of producing healthy, low-cost meals. Four years later the Boston School Committee began receiving meals from the New England Kitchen, and Richards had laid the foundation for a model of what was to eventually become the NSLP.

Philadelphia's first penny lunch program, organized and run by a private charity, began in 1894, and its most significant contribution was the creation of the Lunch Committee of the Home and School League, the precursor to the modern-day Parent Teacher Association (PTA), which was instrumental in expanding the lunch program to nine other area schools.

About a decade later, in New York, Robert Hunter published *Poverty*, in which he made the assertion that between 60,000 and

About 99 percent of today's agricultural production depends on only 24 different domesticated plant species. Of those, rice, wheat, and corn account for most of the world's caloric intake.

> Every year we spend $7 billion on school lunch, $50 billion on diet aids, $115 billion on diet-related illness and more than $200 billion on the war.

70,000 children in New York City arrived at school with empty stomachs. It prompted a firestorm of investigative reports, including John Spargo's *The Bitter Cry of the Children*, published in 1906. Spargo supported Hunter's claims and urged society at large to take action on behalf of the children. Spargo's work in turn spurred further studies by physicians who began publishing reports about the malnutrition of New York City schoolchildren, which later led to a plea from the superintendent of New York City schools, William Maxwell, for a school lunch program where children could purchase healthy, low-cost lunches every day. Maxwell's wishes were granted and two schools were elected to participate in a trial run. Their success was undeniable and two years later the New York City School Board approved the program and opened the door for a citywide school lunch program overseen by physicians with an eye toward honoring the ethnic and cultural traditions of the various school populations. Not surprisingly, the overall health of New York City's schoolchildren showed improvement very quickly. Ten years later, seventeen public schools were participating in the program and the first food safety measures, which included physical exams for food handlers as well as smallpox vaccines, were established. Before the start of the First World War, thirteen states and Washington, D.C., had some type of school food program in place.

As the war began the school lunch program was expanded, due in no small part to the fact that approximately one-third of all young men attempting to enlist were turned away because of diseases attributable to malnutrition. When the Great Depression hit in the 1930s, private charities and individuals could no longer support school food programs and hunger in America became more widespread. It was clear that the federal government would have to step in.

People were hungry, not because there was a shortage of food, but because they didn't have the money to buy food, and, as a result, American farmers were left with enormous agricultural surpluses and were in danger of losing their farms. In an effort to both assist farmers by purchasing their products and feed needy families and schoolchildren, the Congress passed the Agricultural Act of 1935 (Public Law 320) which "required the cooperation of federal, state, and local governments to implement, and establish a structure upon which future commodity distributions programs were built."

During this time the Works Progress Administration (WPA) was organized to provide work on public projects to the unemployed, and school lunches were a perfect fit for the program. Not only did WPA workers cook and serve lunches, but they canned the fresh fruits and vegetables provided to them through the surplus program and through school gardens. By 1941 school lunches were being served by the WPA in every state to a total of about 2 million schoolchildren. The program employed more than 64,000 people in school lunch programs alone at that time. By 1942, 6 million children were participating.

Unfortunately, with the onset of World War II the school lunch program took a hit as surpluses were redirected to feed troops, but in 1943 Congress amended the Agricultural Act of 1935 to "provide school districts directly with funds for implementation of their school lunch programs."

At the war's end, General Lewis Blaine Hershey, director of the Selective Service System, declared that malnutrition was a *national security risk* and stated before Congress that the United States had 155,000 war casualties directly related to malnutrition. It became clear that strong federal legislation was necessary, and in the summer of 1946 the National School Lunch Act (Public Law 396) was signed by President Harry S. Truman. The new law specified permanent funding through the Secretary of Agriculture to:

1. Assist with the health of the nation's children, and
2. Ensure a market for farmers.

With the passing of PL 396, the National School Lunch Program was given an unshakable foundation.

The guidelines for administration of school lunch programs under PL 396 include:

1. Lunches must meet minimum nutritional requirements set by the Secretary of Agriculture.
2. Free or reduced-cost meals must be made available to children whom local authorities determine unable to pay.
3. Discrimination against children unable to pay is forbidden.
4. The program must be operated on a nonprofit basis.
5. Foods designated by the Secretary as abundant must be utilized.
6. Donated commodity foods must be utilized.
7. Records, receipts, and expenditures must be kept and submitted in a report to the state agency when required.

Funds were also set aside specifically for the purchase of equipment so that money given to schools for food would be used only to purchase food. In 1954 the Special Milk Program was set in place, making surplus milk available to schools.

Between 1955 and 1965–1966, a decline in nutritional intake was reported by the Household Food Consumption Survey of 1965–66. Reaction to this discovery resulted in the Child Nutrition Act of 1966 (Public Law 89-642), allowing for increased funding to create programs whose sole purpose was to improve child nutrition. The Special Milk Program became part of the Child Nutrition Act, and through this Act, schools were provided funds for the purchase of equipment. Beginning in 1966, a Pilot Breakfast Program was given a two-year test run and allowances were made for hiring more employees. It was at this point that all school food programs were placed under the aegis of one federal agency, standardizing the management of school lunch programs across the country.

In the 1970s nutritionists began taking a closer look at school meals and criticized the program for not taking age or body types into account. The same meals were being served to all students—athletes, obese children, undernourished kids, first-graders, and high school students alike. They also questioned the general healthfulness of school lunches. After a decade of discussion, new regulations were put in place that, among other things, included a provision that required different portion sizes for children of different age groups.

Also in the 1970s, vending machines made their appearance in public schools. There was some immediate concern at that time as to the types of products being sold. As a result of Secretary of Agriculture issued regulations in 1980 restricting the sale of sodas, gum, and certain types of candy. The regulations were overturned in a 1984 lawsuit brought by the National Soft Drink Association. The judge presiding over the case stated that the Secretary of Agriculture was permitted only to regulate food sales within the cafeteria. So although they were not allowed in cafeterias, vending machines once again found their way onto public school campuses around the country.

The 1980s were a time of great strain on the school lunch program. The Reagan administration forced budget cuts, causing meal prices to rise and some children to drop out of the program altogether. In an effort to save money and still appear to be meeting the federal guidelines for a healthy school lunch, the government made attempts to add certain foods to the permissible list. The one that made the most people sit up and take notice was the shocking allowance of ketchup as a vegetable.

By the time President Clinton took office, the USDA was still falling well short of meeting its own dietary guidelines in the public school system. The fat content of school lunches was well above recommended dietary guidelines, and meals were falling well short of students' needed nutrient values. Ellen Haas was appointed as Assistant Secretary of Agriculture in charge of food and consumer affairs, overseeing the National School Lunch Program. Haas and Secretary of Agriculture Mike Espy held a series of national hearings and put together the School

Most Americans have traces of a half dozen pesticides in their urine.

> Brian Halweil of the Worldwatch Institute reported that every dollar spent with a local food business is worth $2.50 to the community.

Meals Initiative for Healthy Children in the summer of 1994. It required that schools meet USDA Federal Dietary Guidelines by 1998. The directive that an average of 30 percent or less of the week's calorie count come from fat (10 percent from saturated fat) angered major players in the meat and dairy industries who had been particularly reliant upon the school food program to take their surpluses. Nevertheless Haas pushed forward, making her School Meals Initiative the first substantial revision to the National School Lunch Program in nearly 50 years.

In spite of the fact that Haas's proposal became a federal mandate in 1994, schools still struggled to meet its demands. Poultry, soy, and a greater variety of fruits and vegetables have been designated as permissible by the USDA, but fat content is down by only 4 percent and remains at about 34 percent on average. And while 70 percent of all elementary schools meet government-mandated nutrient guidelines, only 20 percent of secondary schools have been able to do so. Worse, more snacks are offered at school than ever before and fast-food chains are slowly but surely inching their way into the school system. Cash-poor schools look to school snacks and fast food to help raise money for extracurricular programs, among other things. Some people assert that while in school, children most often choose the foods they get at home. While that may be true, kids are also being bombarded with extremely persuasive advertising for high-fat, low-nutrient foods every day. Food companies spend approximately $30 billion to underwrite about 40,000 commercials annually. It's nearly impossible for the National School Lunch Program to come out ahead if fast foods are among the choices in the lunchroom. When presented with a familiar Taco Bell selection and school cafeteria mystery meat, it's really a no-brainer what most kids will choose.

School meals reach nearly 27 million kids a day and for some, what they eat at school remains the most nutritious meal of their day, which is great news. Still, the childhood obesity crisis is at an all-time high. Kids are getting fatter and fatter, and it is our job to help them. In addition to helping you learn about good childhood nutrition in a way that allows you to prepare high-quality, nutritious meals for your children at home, this book will also show you how to reach out to your local school lunch administrators to improve the quality of lunches served at your children's schools.*

First Things First: Breakfast

Intuitively most of us just know that poor nutrition isn't good for the body. We can all probably recall a time when we ate poorly and felt sluggish and tired afterward. Other times, when our diets were healthful and varied, our bodies just seemed to work better. Our attention spans were longer, and we felt good. In his work at Massachusetts General Hospital and Harvard Medical School, Dr. J. Michael Murphy has seen proof that what kids eat for breakfast affects their performance in school. Between one-third and one-half of all teenagers skip breakfast, and it's no surprise that with all the rushing around we do to get out the door in the morning, the rates are high even among pre-K and elementary school students. It's hard sometimes to get kids fed when both parents have to be out the door to work early in the morning. But Murphy tells us that his research shows breakfast is an imperative. Children who eat breakfast function better both cognitively and emotionally. He said that "there is a huge body of knowledge, including very many recent studies with large samples, showing that by and large, children who skip breakfast do more poorly on virtually any measure—whether it's standardized test scores, cognitive test scores, nutrition, obesity, or health." The same studies also show that when a high-quality breakfast is served in school, tardiness and absenteeism drop considerably. Some fore-thinking

Whole grains contain fiber, remove toxins, and promote digestive health.

*Demas, Antonia, PhD., *A History of the School Lunch Program*. Food Studies Institute, Inc., Trumansburg, NY, 2000.

schools have taken breakfast one step further and have been making sure that meal is available in the classroom when children arrive in the morning. About this, Murphy added:

> Studies have also been definitive that breakfast in the classroom is twice as powerful as even just a free breakfast in a cafeteria. Part of why it's more difficult in the cafeteria has to do with the logistics of getting hundreds of children in and out of the cafeteria in the morning. Add to that late buses and other unforeseen challenges and many kids just get to school too late to take advantage of the program. Just putting breakfast in the classroom, maybe even on the kids' desks, is a much stronger way of getting them to take advantage of it. It ensures that it's available when kids arrive and it also creates a nice environment in the classroom where people all eat together [and have a sense of community] they wouldn't otherwise experience.

Sadly, not all schools offer a breakfast program, much less breakfast at the kids' desks, but if your child's school does have a breakfast program, keep Dr. Murphy's research in mind—it could make a world of difference.

It Takes a Village—and More

Not only does school lunch reform take a village to implement, it may take a county or an entire region. Much of it depends on local climate, access to farms, and the size of the school system. Because each school is different, each school has a different way of approaching school lunch reform. To give you some ideas about how to implement changes in your children's schools we're highlighting the success stories of a wide range of

---

As dietary fiber increases, the risk of heart disease can fall by as much as 35 percent.

schools and school systems around the country. Our first stop is the school that inspired both of us to start down our individual paths toward large scale school lunch reform: The Ross School in East Hampton, New York.

The Ross School

Located in East Hampton, New York, the Ross School was founded in 1991 by Courtney Ross and Steven J. Ross. When they conceived their original plan for the school, their aspiration was to create an environment and innovative model that would "transform education." Their vision included every aspect of student life, from the school's general atmosphere to curriculum and even school meals.

After our collaboration on *Bitter Harvest*, Ann was approached by Courtney Ross to take the position of executive chef at the school. Ross wanted to improve and expand the school's existing food program, and Ann embraced the unique opportunity to build a high-quality school lunch program. Once at Ross, Ann oversaw the final design and implementation of the school's Café, which includes a wood-fired pizza oven, and hand-picked ceramic dishware, glasses, and silverware. The school's dining room grew into a beautiful space on the second floor, "up in the trees," where children and teachers alike would eat delicious food together in a civilized and relaxed atmosphere. The food itself was cooked fresh for service by trained professional chefs and cooks. There were no steam tables, no reheated foods, and no fried high-fat foods. Ann believed that if she provided flavorful food to kids they would eat it, regardless of its nutritional content. Overwhelmingly the Ross food experience showed that if you put delicious food in front of kids, even if it's vegetables and whole grains, they'll eat it because they're attracted to the flavors. This is the primary reason they love fast food. They don't eat it because they know it's bad for them, they eat it because they like the taste, and fast food has flavor down to a science—literally. Chemists create the flavor additives that make those foods so appealing.

There's been a fear in the field of childhood nutrition that kids will run away from nutritious food, but at Ross, Ann and her staff showed that kids will literally eat tons of vegetables if they taste good. Making them taste good might be as complicated as creating a new recipe around a certain product, or it might simply mean that the vegetable be cooked to perfection by people who know how to cook. With the right staff in place, creating delicious food is easy. Beth Collins, who took over as executive chef after Ann left, told us that she feels

> very fortunate because we have a kitchen filled with chefs; a kitchen filled with people who love food, love flavor, and know how to handle fresh product because it's what they've always done. They come from a restaurant background and I don't think you can really undervalue how much that means to the quality of what happens at this particular place. I think it's really the key factor in putting together the great products we get from farms while trying to prepare great food and educate kids at the same time . . . I think that having a chef involved, particularly somebody who has a really strong relationship to fresh product and is devoted to it is the way to begin these relationships. You really need to have a lot of energy and commitment and passion about it. In this place there is a lot of passion.

The Supply Chain

In having a commitment to local and regional farmers, one of the primary challenges at Ross was setting up the supply chain. It's difficult to create a system that brings in a variety of foods from a large number of sources in a timely manner while keeping spoilage to a minimum and ensuring that the food will be flavorful meal after meal. Without a top-notch supply chain even the best menu in the world will fall short because the product isn't there. Ann and her staff were able to set up high-quality supply chains that consistently delivered top-notch food day after day. In a conscious effort to promote the longevity, or sustainability,

---

Tomatoes are very high in the carotenoid lycopene; eating foods with carotenoids can lower your risk of cancer.

---

of local small businesses, the Ross School relies heavily on small-scale local farmers and has created meaningful, reciprocal relationships with many of their suppliers.

John Halsey is an apple and peach farmer who provides the school with nearly 3,500 gallons of apple cider a year. Collins told us that one of the biggest challenges in engaging local farmers in the supply chain was getting them to understand that "we were serious about buying their products as much as we could and I think once we got past the initial hurdle of yes, we're going to buy your product and yes, we're going to pay you on a timely basis, [the farmers were] really very welcoming at that point."

Halsey agrees that he was reluctant to take on the challenge of selling to Ross at first even though he admits that it's easier for a farmer to sell to a school, church, or other institution than to scale down and attempt to sell products direct to the consumer as many small farms are doing these days. An arrangement like the one he has with Ross is ideal. For him, cider is a good fit because it allows him to turn his second-quality fruit into a good product. In fact, for schools like Ross smaller farms are a better choice, because large farms may not be able to adapt to the smaller, high-quality needs of schools. The 3,500 gallons Halsey supplies annually would be, as Halsey says,

> a tiny drop in the bucket in commercial food production and packaging in the U.S. When we talk about supplying schools or small businesses we have to remember that farmers in general in this country are supplying King Kongs, and so 3,500 gallons of cider is a sizable amount for us, but a cider mill that's turning out 3,500 gallons an hour wouldn't think of it as much business.

When Ross first approached him, Halsey looked at the school like every other customer he had. He took the job, made every effort to

EECO Farm

by Beth Collins, Executive Chef, The Ross School

Getting your hands dirty is the ultimate entree into understanding what ends up on your plate. I had done a little gardening prior to moving from New York City to the more rural environment of East Hampton, New York, but I had no idea how gardening would become a cornerstone of my existence here. I know now that I will forever be a gardener.

At the Ross School where I work I've tended our 13-box kitchen garden since its inception in the spring of 2002. I love that garden. It's nice and tidy with its twelve 4×8 raised beds and an octagonal bed in the center as the focal point. I've spread it beyond the boxes, adding compost to the sandy ground along the south wall, planting sunflowers and cosmos to bring color to the edges. The boxes have been home to an abundance of "crops" from asparagus to zinnias. But with all its beauty and accessibility to the back door of the Café, my passion for it pales in comparison to my other garden suitor, the two 20×20-foot beds I've planted for the last three seasons at the East End Community Organic Farm (EECO).

What is the difference? Isn't it all the same stuff—seeds, soil, sun, food crops, and flowers? "Kind of" would be my answer. In the Ross School Café, on a daily basis we "teach" local food and sustainable food choices by serving wonderful meals. We demonstrate where our food comes from by using great locally grown organic product. As wonderful as that sounds, it is a struggle to truly teach what agriculture means in our daily lives. The labor associated with a single potato is tough to translate until you've gone out in a field and dug them yourself.

EECO Farm was established as a nonprofit organization four years ago with a mission to demonstrate and teach methods of sustainable agriculture. It began on 42 acres of land leased from the Town of East Hampton. Through the creative work of the founding executive directors Lauren Jarrett and Annie Bliss, the town took the unlikely path of believing an organic farm was a better choice for the town than soccer fields, and EECO Farm's journey began.

There was nothing on this land but compacted soil, tired from a hundred years of conventional potato farming. Four years later EECO Farm is far more than that. It is a vibrant collection of families of the East End who have taken a turn at "farming" a 20×20 plot. Based on the English concept of public gardens, EECO

Farm began its first season with 45 community garden plots, a few acres of production-row farming and a lot of enthusiasm. This year they hosted more than a hundred families and had eighteen acres under production for their roadside farm stand, farmers' market sales, and wholesale sales. In season the farm hosts scores of local schools, has weekly seminars ranging from soil science to making pickles, and has a monthly full-moon potluck for the members and community at large.

In the most popular summer destination in the New York metro area, tending your garden at a summer sunset in the middle of EECO Farm is the best experience available in the Hamptons. People who have never sowed a seed find pleasure and success in "farming" in a full-sun environment that is rarely found in most backyard gardens. The community is full of real farmers like Dale Haubrich, who leases an acre on the property and brings volumes of experience to the table, happily passing on the best way to grow corn organically, or diagnosing why your cabbage isn't forming just right. A walk around the community garden plots is a lesson in the diversity of gardening approaches when observing something as mundane as trellising peas. [The plots may be more "farm" looking like mine, or have paths and mounds and tomato teepees.] Some gardeners are even trying their hand at growing wine grapes.

There is a vigor brought by the scores of individuals coming together at EECO Farm, some of whom are veterans of gardening and some who are discovering it for the first time. For those of us who have participated in the growth of the farm from borrowing water from the neighboring nursery to having both a well and electricity this year, there's a certain proud parent feeling—you are waving the flag of EECO Farm and knowing your garden is more than simply growing the best tomatoes. Your tomatoes were grown without chemicals, you see how the soil in your bed is changing from that bedrock lifeless dirt of the first season to the fluffy loam of this year, and somehow organic and local food takes on a new life. You start dreading winter with the prospect of shopping the produce aisle at the grocery store, knowing there is no local organic produce there.

But in the dead of winter you can dream of next summer when the outstretched hands of the open field at EECO Farm speaks volumes—with your feet planted firmly in the warm soil you dream of seeds and water becoming your food and best of all, the community that is EECO Farm.

Numerous vegetables are high in carotenoids, such as carrots, spinach, sweet potatoes, and collard greens.

meet the client's needs, and was cautiously optimistic about making any major changes to his business. Because the Ross School was "very, very definite to their commitment to local agriculture and business," Halsey felt more comfortable making changes to meet the school's needs and has worked out a system of delivery that doesn't require the school to have storage available for large quantities of cider.

Halsey has 70 acres with 20 in production for apples, and 4 in production for peaches. He grows about 10,000 bushels of apples a year. It's been relatively easy for him to work with Ross because the school wants a high-quality product and is willing to pay for it. He told us that

> there are businesses that are not as apt to pay for quality and this is what we run into with the public school systems. We [work with schools on that] and we do sell to a couple of public school systems, but they are not nearly as concerned about quality as they are about cost. Quite often they will buy a lower-quality product off the open market or a government-supported product . . . I do think the future is bright for small farmers like me who want to produce and supply a service to institutions, especially if parents get involved in the food supply to their children.

Putting the Lesson in Lunch

At Ross they're not just talking about creating a healthy plate of food, they make food an ongoing part of the school's curriculum. The day we interviewed Chef Collins, the sixth grade was studying ancient Greece as part of the Ross School's integrated curriculum. For their part, the kitchen staff did some research into the kinds of foods that were typical in ancient Greece and then developed a menu around them. Part of the menu included a piece that would allow the kids some hands-on kitchen time, so that afternoon there were twenty 11- and 12-year-olds rolling grape leaves while the kitchen staff educated them about the acidic properties of the leaves and the importance of pickling as a method of food preservation in ancient Greece. The same students were there during that day's lunch service, bringing the experience full circle for both students and staff.

For Ann, one of the true joys of working at the Ross School was participating in the fully integrated curriculum. When the students were studying the Renaissance, the kitchen staff prepared a Renaissance feast for them. During the period of study that included India, executive sous-chef Deena Chafetz put together a spice tasting for the students. It was that spice tasting that led to one of Ann's favorite Ross moments. Some of the sixth graders were in the Café where they were speaking to Mrs. Ross, who asked what they were learning. They'd just come from the spice tasting and were enthusiastically telling her about what they'd just done. They told her they were glad the spice tasting was happening at that time and not the previous year. When Ross asked why they replied, "Because our palates have grown so much since last year. We can taste so much better now."

While there are concrete food and nutrition lessons, much of the teaching at Ross happens passively, meaning the children are given lots of choices, but they're all healthy choices. They begin to understand by example what is healthy for them. Collins admits that it can be a challenge at times because

the kids can still derail [the school's intentions] somehow. They'll take a plate of rice and then go back to the pasta and don't take their vegetable. It's important to remember that just putting good product out there doesn't finish the job. You have to continue to interact with the children, and you can't give up because you're met with some initial resistance. You have to understand that they change very much from the beginning of the year to the end of the year and then even more from one grade to the next. One year, for example, you'll have one kid who doesn't eat much and the next they eat a wide variety of things. They may backslide the following year and stop eating certain things again. The interaction with the kids is really important. You know, really trying to create a dialogue with them around the food that's positive so that they don't feel like eating vegetables is a job they have to do.

Collins believes that it is beneficial to involve and educate the parents as well because they can help support the school's initiative at home. And they may even learn something themselves. Early in the school year the parents of Ross School students are invited to a meeting held in conjunction with the Parents' Association, during which the kitchen staff does a presentation about the school's food program with the campus registered dietician, Hailey London (who helped Ann create the Healthy Kid's Meal Wheel). They let them know what types of foods will be appearing on the school lunch menu, which changes daily, enabling them to have informed conversations about it with their children. Collins asserts that parents are "really important in the whole equation," and believes that giving them the tools to communicate with their children about food allows them to make better use of the limited time they do have around meals and food in general.

The Ross School has raised the bar on school food in a number of other ways, too. The Café is located in the Wellness Center and all of the Ross students participate in physical activities every day. From soccer to basketball to yoga and weight training, Ross has made fitness an integral part of the day. Hailey London plays a consistent role in the lives of Ross School children as well. She worked collaboratively with Ann and Beth, and teaches the students about nutrition, health, and sustainability, and actually grades the students on what they have for lunch and what they know about their food choices. At

Calories on the rise: In the 1960s a McDonald's small fries was 210 calories, versus 610 calories today for a large.

Ross, cooking is a graduation requirement, and the students all work in the school's garden or on one of the local farms like Quail Hill or EECO Farm.

New York City

The Ross School isn't far from New York City in distance, but it is light years away from the New York City Public Schools' lunch program in virtually every possible way. Cooper's experience at Ross, though different, gave her the tools to work with some of the most inspired and inspiring people involved in New York City's massive school lunch program reform. Home to the largest, most complex lunch program in the country, New York City hosts a system that feeds more than 860,000 kids daily and it is undergoing some striking changes.

CookShop and the SchoolFood Plus Initiative

In the 1990s, New York law mandated that public schools must purchase food from the lowest bidder, a practice that frequently resulted in the consumption of low-quality food by New York City schoolchildren. Toni Liquori, of Teachers College, Columbia University, and former senior program manager at FoodChange, a hunger and food advocacy group in New York City, was alarmed by this practice and believed that poor quality food contributed to the overall poor health of the district's children. The way she saw it, their health was being sold to the lowest bidder and she was determined to make changes. It was at that time that she conceived CookShop, a lower/elementary school–based nutrition education program that teaches children about food, flavor, and nutrition through hands-on discovery. Mindful of the underlying concepts of eating all parts of the plant (root, stem, leaves, flower, fruit, and seed), choosing regionally-grown fruits and vegetables when possible, and focusing the curriculum on foods that school foodservice staff have access to through their procurement system, the CookShop staff chose the following—broccoli/cauliflower, rice, corn, wheat, apples, collards, carrots, beans, lettuce, and potatoes. CookShop gives the children access to unprocessed whole foods they may never have seen or tasted before and exposes them, many for the first time, to agriculture. Its goal is to increase children's consumption of whole and minimally processed fruits, vegetables, legumes, and whole grains with an interdisciplinary approach that includes vocabulary, natural science, home economics, and math. The program has been implemented in New York City's low-income neighborhoods where the incidences of malnutrition and childhood obesity are generally highest.

In the classroom, children become food explorers. During the month they study apples, for example, they start out by reading a letter from a real apple farmer, after which they break into small groups and do hands-on exploration. They examine the apple's skin, the core, the stem, and they talk about apple trees. There are posters and sequence cards to show growth from seed to mature plant and they study what the apple tree looks like throughout the seasons. There is always a tasting. For apples the children try four different varieties and talk about how they taste, comparing them one to the other, in an exercise that helps them develop descriptive food adjectives that will allow them to have a conversation about their apple experience. Eventually they graduate from apple explorers to apple chefs and prepare a standardized recipe for applesauce. Each of the ten foods is taught in the same way.

Karen Wadsworth, a former FoodChange employee who worked with Liquori on CookShop, reported that an evaluation of the program showed that the more children are exposed to a food, the more they are likely to taste it and adopt it as a regular part of their diet. There is no doubt in our minds that magical things happen when children have a hand in preparing their food. All of a sudden they're trying foods they never thought they'd like, which leads them to become more independent food explorers in their lives outside of school.

A small Coke in the 1960s was 80 calories (8.5 ounces), versus 250 calories for a large (20-ounce) one today.

The Dirt-to-Plate Connection

Wadsworth told us that often what is lacking in an urban setting is the direct connection to the farm. When asked where food comes from the vast majority of urban children reply with a hearty "the grocery store!" In an effort to overcome this barrier, CookShop showcases regional farmers with letters written by the farmers along with pictures of them, their farms, and their products. Not only does this connection help the kids by teaching them about healthy food choices, but it increases the purchasing of regional farm products by schools. In fact the school system's featured apple farmer, Joy Crist, is just one of many who have found a new market for their products. The apple slices that are being served in the New York City public schools come, in part, from her farm. Having the schools as a secure market even gave another farmer, Jerry Digert, the confidence to extend himself and build a processing plant that would allow the farmer to slice and bag the apples directly for the school.

CookShop is supported by CookShop Cafeteria, which encourages food service staff to cook and serve minimally processed plant-based foods, and the CookShop Food and Fitness Council, which "guides the establishment of health committees in the New York City school system."

During the 2005/2006 school year, CookShop began running in 15 schools and is currently in 100 schools.

CookShop inspired a collaboration of the city's departments of Education and Health, the State's Department of Agriculture and Markets, Columbia Teachers College, and a local community advocacy organization, FoodChange, to create SchoolFood Plus, the goal of which is to "improve both childhood nutrition and the State's agricultural economy." Government workers, community advocates, and educators work, as Kate Adamick, former senior program officer of the

Department of Defense (DoD) and DoDFresh

The Department of Defense (DoD) is the largest food-service provider in the United States. It originally served military bases and installations around the country, but expanded in the early- and mid-1990s to include hospitals, schools, and prisons. In 1995 it launched DoDFresh as a pilot program designed to increase the purchasing of fresh American-grown produce by public schools around the country.

DoDFresh distributes fresh fruits and vegetables purchased from U.S. farms to schools that use Department of Defense Fair Share Entitlement dollars as designated in the 2002 Farm Bill, as well as commodity allocations, to procure their produce. In the program's first year, eight states participated in DoDFresh and fresh produce valued in excess of $3.25 million was purchased by schools. The program was so well-received that the following year all states were invited to participate. DoDFresh spending by schools increased annually and was up to $25 million during the 2002 school year. After the 2002 Farm Bill passed, spending shot up to $50 million in 2003 and remains that high in 2006. As of this writing, forty-three states plus Washington, D.C., Puerto Rico, the Virgin Islands, and Guam are taking part in this groundbreaking program.

Through DoDFresh, states and individual schools have access to nearly 900 items including fresh lettuces, mushrooms, broccoli, apples, pears, oranges, melons, strawberries, pineapples, greens (collards and kale, among others), avocados, tomatoes, peaches, cucumbers, carrots, and bananas. Thus far, program participants have been very happy with the variety and quality of the food they receive.

In New York City, more than 3 million dollars of fresh produce is coming through DoDFresh. Since the CookShop recipes use regionally grown produce, we are beginning to see movement within DoDFresh to source and deliver a regionally based product in New York, a trend that will hopefully increase in other parts of the country.

A McDonald's hamburger in the 1960s was 250 calories, versus today's Big Extra at 810.

SchoolFood Plus Initiative told us, "behind the scenes . . . to develop new plant-based recipes, implement higher nutrition standards for prepared foods, strategize new ways in which to procure more fresh foods from local farmers, and struggle to overcome the very real hurdles of limited budgets, ill-equipped kitchens, and undermanned cooking staffs."

The heart of the SchoolFood Plus program is thirty-two recipes based on the ten regionally grown fruits, vegetables, and legumes from the CookShop program that are being served three times a week in seventy schools and weekly in all 1,200 schools in New York City. To those who don't know how enormous the New York City school system is this may not seem like a lot, but it's huge. At least once a week—more often for some—all 860,000 children in New York City public schools are being served a healthy, delicious plant-based lunch item that's been prepared with food grown in the region. Considering the scale, this alone is an awe-inspiring accomplishment.

But there's more. The originators of CookShop and the SchoolFood Plus Initiative believe that positive change hinges on a broader education of the entire school community. While the school works to implement CookShop's standards and ideals "councils, coalitions, and networks of concerned teenagers, parents, educators, healthcare professionals, and community advocates gather to improve food and fitness in individual schools, to support and challenge the department of education's ongoing efforts to improve school food system-wide, and to harness the collective power of other large urban school districts across the country to affect change in both food industry practice and federal nutrition policy," Adamick told us.

The school system's primary concerns are "increasing awareness through education, changing institutional practices, and creating community interest in and support for better school food." We believe that if that kind of change can take place in the second largest (Department of Defense being the largest) food-service provider in America, every school district in this country can make similar changes using Cook-Shop and the SchoolFood Plus Initiative as a model.

E.A.T.W.I.S.E. Kids

At Park West High School in New York City, there is one incredible group of teens working to improve their health and eating habits as well as those of their friends, neighbors, and relatives. Known as E.A.T.W.I.S.E. (Educated and Aware Teens Who Inspire Smart Eating), Rosalba Nueva, Alexandra Munoz, Juan Torres, Ashley Guzman, Jesse Asencio, and Isreal Jackson originally came together in an after-school program with the goal of learning to incorporate healthier eating habits into their daily lives and their school cafeteria. The elective after-school program, run by FoodChange staffers at Park West, was designed as a program to help the students understand good nutrition and food choices. Over time it has grown into this student-run program, which continues to be supported by FoodChange staff.

Before getting involved in E.A.T.W.I.S.E. these kids ate junk and fast food constantly. They tell us that on the streets junk food is referred to as "snack crack" because of the sugar high they get from eating it. When they began their work with E.A.T.W.I.S.E., they tasted fruits, vegetables, fruit snacks, and non-soda beverages—a far cry from everything they'd been eating, school lunch included. As the students began learning about healthy food choices, and tasting the new foods, they came to understand that they could control what they put in their bodies. It suddenly clicked with them how important that was.

As the program progressed and their eating habits improved they began to realize they were feeling better and doing better at school and in sports. One student reported that he was faster in his track-and-field events when he ate good food.

Even though physically they could feel the benefits of the program, it wasn't always easy. In some cases their social lives suffered. Before

Refined carbohydrates react like sugar in the body, lowering immune systems, spiking insulin, creating cravings and feeding candida yeast, which often causes allergies and intolerances.

> Whole grains help prevent diabetes and cancer by stabilizing blood sugar—three servings daily reduces the risk of developing high blood sugar by 27 percent.

E.A.T.W.I.S.E. they would go to McDonald's after school with their friends and, after sporting events, entire teams would meet there to eat and hang out. As they've changed their views on food and eating, these kids have also changed their social scenes. They have such passion about their work with E.A.T.W.I.S.E. that they chose it over some friends and activities—which we all know is saying a lot, because the teenage social scene normally takes precedence over all else, no matter how difficult it may be for some children to keep up. We think this development alone could be viewed as remarkable enough, but these kids have also made changes at home, which has been a challenge as well because their new-found health consciousness hasn't always been embraced by their families who were happy with the status quo and had no desire to change.

One young woman, Ashley, told us that she struggles with her dad, saying that "he's like, 'You just eat the food that we give you,' but I want to grow up and have my body healthy. I don't want to end up dying at an early age and I keep telling him and telling him, 'You know I still need you, Dad, you're overweight and you just got type 2 diabetes and I don't want you to die or anything,' and he's like, 'I'm still gonna eat my fried chicken and rice and beans,' and I'm like, 'Dad, please!' and we struggle with that." Other kids have had similar experiences, but they have persevered and made changes on their own, even without family support.

Some actually have managed to inspire their families to take on the challenge of changing their lifestyle. Ashley went on to say that she used to live in Puerto Rico and she ate all three meals at McDonald's—every day. Her doctor warned that she was overweight. When she became involved with E.A.T.W.I.S.E. she started eating more healthfully. Within two months she had lost forty pounds and realized just how beneficial the program was for her. She exercises now and continues to maintain a healthy diet, dropping nearly fifty pounds total. She believes that she has actually gained friends because of her weight loss, and her family was so

Healthy fats include omega-3 fatty acids, monounsaturated, and polyunsaturated fats, which are found in corn, soybean, safflower, fish, and cottonseed. All of these healthy fats lower LDL and raise HDL.

impressed with her efforts that they started making changes. Even her grandmother, who ate a lot of fried foods, adopted some changes when her granddaughter began engaging her in conversation about food choices and brought home some recipes to try. Now she eats salads, fresh fruits, and vegetables, and chooses healthier cooking methods. Another young woman, Alexandra, told us that she and her mother began shopping at the farmers' market as a result of the program and it has blossomed into a mother–daughter bonding experience for them. They get up early and head out for a leisurely morning, looking at and choosing fresh, wholesome, and oftentimes new and interesting foods. They enjoy it much more than a boring trip to the grocery store.

In an effort to raise awareness, the E.A.T.W.I.S.E. kids have hosted healthy smoothie sales at Park West and have begun conducting meetings with other students to bring health and nutrition information to students at their school and beyond.

Promise Academy

Promise Academy, a charter school, is part of the Harlem Children's Zone (HCZ), which was founded in 1970 as a nonprofit community-based organization working to improve the quality of life for kids and families in some of New York City's toughest, most run-down neighborhoods. In all, there are fifteen HCZ centers in New York that serve nearly 13,000 people, 8,600 of whom are at-risk children. Their work focuses on everything from education to recreation and their purpose is to rebuild the community life in each neighborhood where they have a presence. In late summer of 2004, Toni Liquori, Hiram Bonner, and FoodChange (formerly Community Food Resource Center) along with the Kellogg Foundation, collaborated on the Harlem S.O.U.L. (Sustainable, Organic, Uptown,

Local) Food Project, which facilitates a connection between New York's low-income residents and regional farmers. While Promise Academy's kitchens were being built, farm-fresh products were being prepared in FoodChange's Harlem kitchen under the direction of executive chef Andrew Benson and delivered daily to the students of Promise. In early 2005, Chef Benson and his staff moved to the Promise kitchens.

Benson began his school food-service career working as a chef in one of New York City's public schools where he was disturbed by the dearth of quality food. At Promise, where most everything is cooked from scratch, Benson believes that the food, while only marginally more costly, is far superior to anything found in the city's public school cafeterias. Students aren't accustomed to eating fresh, whole foods, and Benson told us that they often come through the line complaining that they won't eat certain things. He handles that problem by putting a little of everything on each student's tray, asking them to at least try it. They often do and are surprised to find they like it. One of Benson's favorite stories is of a couple of kids who had never had fresh broccoli and were afraid to try it. They did and later came back to tell him that it "was the most amazing thing." They were thrilled.

There are many success stories in the Promise food program, not the least of which is the salad bar. Almost all of the students take something from the salad bar every day and the great thing about it is that virtually all of the ingredients are fresh. Students enjoy it so much that they often argue over who gets to serve salads.

As with other Kellogg-funded programs, Promise's food is based as much as possible in local agriculture. Benson is perhaps proudest of his milk program. He worked with Ronnybrook, a local dairy, to procure their milk, butter, and yogurt and, as a special summertime treat, even ice cream, and told us that his delicious, locally produced milk costs a mere 2/100ths of a cent more per serving than the less tasty, less healthful brand-name version. It's also wonderful to expose students to a food

---

Sources of omega-3 fatty acids include such cold-water fish as cod, salmon, herring, fluke, mackerel, and albacore tuna.

New Jersey Fights Fat Statewide

There is a new set of rules in New Jersey schools. It is, in fact, the boldest school food initiative attempted to date. By September 2007, there will no longer be french fries, soda, candy, and other high-fat foods available to students from pre-K through high school. Anything listing sugar as its first ingredient is a goner, and the only beverages allowed for service will be milk, water, and 100 percent fruit or vegetable juices. No items containing more than 8 grams of fat will be available and beverages other than water and low-fat milk will be limited to serving sizes of less than 12 ounces. There are 600 school districts in New Jersey. This is an enormous and unprecedented undertaking, especially because it addresses high school lunches, which are typically regarded as too difficult and/or controversial for these types of programs.

In 2004 President Bush signed the Child Nutrition and WIC Reauthorization Act, which requires all schools participating in the federal school-meal program to establish wellness policies by 2006. By the end of 2005 New Jersey had jumped way ahead of the federal requirements.

Some schools are already offering baked foods rather than fried, more fruits and vegetables are being made available to kids regularly, hot dogs are made from turkey rather than beef, and smaller dessert items with lower fat contents are being served. School food-service directors caution that these changes have been made slowly and with baby steps—none of this happened overnight. And the kids didn't take to all the changes right away, either. For a lot of these kids, school lunch had been like a snack food free-for-all and it's hard for them to give that up. Nowadays what they're getting in school is comparable to what they find in their cabinets and refrigerators at home. But even though they may be greeting the school changes with resistance, they have adjusted quickly.

Requiring some schools (about 150 of them) to participate in a program called "Shape It Up," created at Rutgers University in conjunction with New Jersey elementary school students, has helped move things along a little more quickly. The program uses interactive projects to illustrate the effects of poor eating habits and teaches kids how to make healthy food choices, even in a fast-food setting.

product that is produced not 100 miles from where they live. Our hope is that other schools will look to schools like Promise for inspiration and begin taking small steps toward overall change and better student health.

Because Promise is an urban school in the heart of Harlem, there is a high demographic probability for behavioral problems. We believe that building a sense of community through food and eating is an essential part of the equation in establishing a more wide-reaching sense of decorum among the students. Adult participation is key and, at Promise, the teachers, principal, and often even the superintendent eat with the students in the cafeteria. In our experience the socialization that occurs at a table of children and adults helps make the cafeteria a place of sharing and encourages a sense of calm and propriety. Allowing the students to see teachers as human beings who eat, think, and socialize outside the classroom helps develop more positive relationships among the students and staff members; giving the teachers a chance to see students in a more relaxed social setting often leads to greater insight into the students' personal lives, which ultimately leads to better student–teacher relationships as well.

Not only does Promise serve wonderful meals at lunch, it also provides students with universal breakfast. For many children, especially in the more disadvantaged areas of our country, school meals may be the healthiest (if not the only!) food they eat in a given day. HCZ's founder Geoffrey Canada, believes that feeding every child during the school day is as important as supplying their books and supplies. In other words, school food is an essential part of every child's educational experience.

Appleton, Wisconsin

Wisconsin's Appleton Central Alternative School (ACAS) has successfully integrated "food smarts" into the curriculum. A partnership with

The National School Lunch Program serves more than 26 million children in over 97,000 schools daily, with a price tag of approximately $7 billion.

Natural Ovens Bakery of Manitowoc has enabled the school system to provide meals of nonchemically processed foods that are low in fat, salt, and sugar, as well as fresh fruits and vegetables. Since this successful program began, teachers and administrators credit this new school lunch curriculum for the exceptional improvements in child behavior and well-being. In fact, the school has been able to quantifiably document:

- Increased ability to concentrate in the school setting (more on-task behavior)
- Increased cognitive development
- Ability to think more clearly, objectively, and rationally
- Fewer health complaints, such as headaches, stomachaches, general malaise
- Increased attendance
- Fewer disciplinary referrals
- Reduced feeling of hunger in mid-morning and/or mid-afternoon
- Less moodiness and more calmness
- Increased practice of good nutrition outside of school

To accomplish these outcomes, ACAS serves both a healthful and nutritious breakfast and lunch. Vending machines have been removed from the confines of the school, and children are not allowed to partake of carry-in food or beverages from outside establishments. Bottled water is available to everyone, and kids are encouraged to carry water bottles. The school reports that an absolutely unprecedented 95 percent of the students at ACAS choose to participate.

According to a publication produced by Natural Ovens Bakery, the breakfast program consists of the following items:

- Bottled water, 100 percent juice, skim milk, and a blended energy drink. The energy drink is made fresh daily with a variety of fruits, juices, and Natural Oven's flax-based energy drink powder (with omega-3s)
- A variety of whole-grain bagels, breads, and muffins—all of

> Only 2 percent of school-age children eat a diet that meets the Food Guide Pyramid's recommendations for all five food groups.

which are free of additives, dyes, artificial preservatives, and saturated fats
- Granola cereal
- Fresh peanut butter, natural fruit preserves, Promise margarine
- Fresh fruits, including bananas, apples, pears, oranges, plums, and other seasonal fruits

The lunch program includes the following:

- Bottled water, 100 percent juice, skim milk, and a blended energy drink.

Appleton Central Alternative School's Six Components to a Healthy School Nutrition Environment

- A commitment to nutrition and physical activity
- Quality school meals
- Only healthy food choices (variety)
- Pleasant eating environment
- Nutrition education
- Marketing

Every school concerned with changing the way its students eat should pay heed to these six fundamentals for creating a healthier nutrition program. Ann's own experience at the Ross School showed that each one is of equal importance when making widespread changes and not one should be overlooked or left out of the equation.

- A variety of whole-grain bagels, breads, and muffins—all of which are free of additives, dyes, artificial preservatives, and saturated fats
- Salad bar: dark green lettuce (no iceberg head lettuce), cherry tomatoes, carrot sticks, cucumber slices, sliced mushrooms, black olives, peanuts, sunflower seeds, broccoli and cauliflower florets, shredded carrots, diced boiled eggs, croutons made from whole-grain breads, homemade applesauce, shredded cabbage, peach and pear slices, pineapple chunks, and fruit salad.
- Hot entrée: Central offers no à la carte items. Two on-site cooks prepare the meals daily, and no food is prepared by frying in a grease product. One meat- and one plant-based entree are offered daily. Meat products used include lean pork, chicken, turkey, and fish (no beef). A variety of spices, soymilk products, and tofu are used as natural flavor enhancers in many of the recipes. Because [the school participates] in the National School Lunch Program (NSLP), it needs to offer milk; however, no other dairy products are utilized. In addition, it qualifies for and receives federal commodities, selecting only offerings that are nutritious and not heavily processed.

A big part of the program's success is the result of the school district's partnership with Natural Ovens Bakery. We sat down with Melissa Luedtke, the Peak Performance Farm Coordinator at Natural Ovens Bakery for their Nutritional Research Foundation. The foundation was the brainchild of Paul and Barbara Stitch, the owners of Natural Ovens, who wanted to educate young people about nutritious eating and how food affects their behavior. Through the Peak Performance Program they donated bagels and an energy drink mix to select schools so that each child could have a bagel a day. After significant improvements in

56 percent of 8-year-olds and 83 percent of 14-year-olds consume soda every day.

behavior and academics were documented at ACAS, Paul and Barbara put together the school's current breakfast and lunch program.

The program's overwhelming success led Natural Ovens Bakery to look at working with other area schools on developing similar programs. The bakery still only provides the baked goods, but also supplies each school with a menu and instructions on how to prepare foods and work with vendors to procure the healthful foods necessary to implement the Natural Ovens menu.

The bakery also gives schools a seventy-five-page packet featuring recipes, menus, vending options, and contact information. An included DVD shows how the program has worked and how students and teachers have been affected by the positive changes there. The entire package costs a mere $25. It can be ordered by contacting Melissa Luedtke, Nutritional Resource Foundation, P.O. Box 730 Manitowoc, WI 54221-0730; phone (920) 758-2500, extension 131.

The program costs ACAS only a fifty cents more per student per day, including the cost of labor. So, if ACAS was spending $2 per child on food, they're now spending $2.50 per child. A 25 percent increase has literally changed these children's lives. Their academic abilities have increased, behavioral problems have decreased, and athletics and attendance have both increased. One of the things we found interesting is that these changes have also saved money in other areas, offsetting the aforementioned increases. Luedtke stressed to us that not every school will be able to make all of the changes they recommend at once, but that even one or two changes will be a significant improvement in children's lives.

Santa Monica/Malibu Unified School District

Each school district has its own unique way of facilitating healthy changes in the school lunch program. Dona Richwine is a nutrition specialist for the Santa Monica/Malibu Unified School District. In early 2005 she sat down to talk with us about the school's Farmers' Market

Salad Bar Program, which was initiated in 1997 by a parent who wanted schools to offer healthier foods at lunch—particularly in the area of produce. The school's food-service director at that time had a lot of doubt about the salad bar program, but he was willing to try it at McKinley Elementary during a summer school program. It was so successful that he opted to initiate the program during the regular school year immediately thereafter. It took several years to get salad bars in all the schools, but today all fourteen are fully operational and are enjoyed fully by one-third of the student body who participate in the school lunch program.

Virtually all the produce, as its name suggests, comes from local farmers' markets. Richwine said, "Occasionally we'll use other things if we get an offering from USDA or something we might have left over from the hot lunch line, like say they have leftover apples, but basically we are a true farm-to-school program." School food-service providers don't actually go to the markets every week because even though it's a small school district, relatively speaking, it would be too time-consuming. Instead, the district sets up a purchasing system at the beginning of the school year whereby a purchasing agent is able to order produce for the entire district from preapproved farmers over the telephone. On Saturdays and Wednesdays a driver retrieves the orders and transports them to the school district's central kitchen where the food is stored temporarily (at most a day or two) prior to distribution to the individual schools. The salad bar coordinators work three very labor-intense hours cutting, washing, chopping, serving, and cleaning. It's a challenge for them to do everything they need to do in their three-hour shift, but because costs could get out of hand on the labor front, a tight rein is kept on the salad bar shifts. Richwine told us that even with the labor, the school district estimates costs to be the same as the regular hot lunch and noted that the salad bars aren't just a component of school lunch, they are an actual hot lunch choice that includes pasta or bread, a protein, and milk.

The most success has been seen in the district's elementary schools, because once the children get to middle and high school they have more choices or they can actually leave campus for lunch.

Richwine told us that although there haven't been any official stud-

> Twenty years ago boys consumed twice as much milk as soda—today they consume twice as much soda as milk.

ies to quantify it, they get a lot of positive feedback from the parents, who love the program. She asserted that "no one would ever dare try to take [the Farmer's Market Salad Bar Program] away from the schools because it's so highly regarded. Everybody really likes it. I have parents who tell me their children eat salad every day." The schools support the salad bar program with nutrition education that is available to teachers on a voluntary basis. Parents of the children who have participated in the schools' nutrition education classes report that their kids are more likely to ask for milk and fresh fruits and vegetables at home as well.

The farmers also believe in the program, which Richwine says is only in part due to the fact that the school district is a fairly large customer. Spending nearly $400 every Wednesday with the same farmer can't hurt. She told us that the farmers are "so committed to the program that they give us discounts and no one has ever raised a price in all the years" she's overseen operation of the salad bar program. The schools don't get the very best of all the crops, but might get seconds on things like apples and citrus—still, the quality is very high and both the school district and the farmers benefit from the exchange, which is the key component in the farm-to-school equation. Without the salad bar program in the Santa Monica/Malibu Unified School District, kids would be limited to choosing from a menu that includes all the standard school lunch fare—hot dogs, pizza, chicken nuggets, and cheeseburgers—and they'd be getting food that was actually cooked by school food-service workers twice a week at most.

The Edible Schoolyard

Chelsea Chapman is the director of Alice Waters' Edible Schoolyard at King Middle School in Berkeley, California. This nationally acclaimed program was the inspiration for a movement that calls for putting gardens in all of California's schools as an across-the-board rethinking of the city's school food program. The garden is a beautiful, lush oasis. Watching the students work in the garden, cook in the kitchen, and eat the fruits of their labor is a joyous experience for teachers, parents, and even just passersby. But there is so much more to it than what is seen by casual observation.

The Edible Schoolyard program is literally at the heart of the King Middle School experience. Farming is cyclic and there is ritual in the act of growing food. Every year one of the first things sixth graders do is harvest the corn planted in the summer by the previous year's outgoing sixth graders. They walk into the field where the cornstalks stand well above their heads. Many of them have never seen corn in its natural state before harvest, and just standing there amid the corn plants is a very powerful experience. Each child picks his own ear of corn and will likely be shocked to find a worm hiding behind the silks. (The garden is organic, so pests are a natural part of the process.) This early discovery gives teachers a jumping-off point for a discussion of pests and the chemicals used in conventional farming. They show the children how to cut out the wormy bit, and then cook the ears in the Edible Schoolyard's outdoor oven. Learning is accomplished through a process as natural and organic as the corn they have picked and for many this first lesson in agriculture is mind-blowingly intense. Right away, they're hooked.

After ten weeks in the garden, the students move into the kitchen where everything really comes together for them. Some of the crops they planted in the fall are ready for harvest and their first big event is the winter squash and end-of-season tomato harvest. This is a significant event because it marks the first time the students will cook. Each grade level is structured similarly, with the students rotating between the garden and the kitchen until they've experienced all growing and harvesting seasons.

---

43 percent of elementary schools, 74 percent of middle schools, and more than 98 percent of high schools provide a variety of unhealthy snack options in vending machines.

The National Cancer Institute spends $1 million annually on the 5-a-Day media campaign, while the soft drink industry spends more than 600 times that marketing their products (most often to children).

More than a decade old now, The Edible Schoolyard has created a true sense of community in the school, which has varied ethnic and financial demographics. One of the most interesting and inspiring outcomes of this program is that it has been a great equalizer. No matter where the students come from, no matter their economic background, they all come to the garden and the kitchen and do the same work together as a team. Chapman told us that in the student evaluations at the end of the year, one of the things that appears consistently is that they are happy to have learned to work with other classmates with whom they had not had any interaction before. There are Latino students who have worked in kitchens (or whose parents have worked in kitchens) and are the most skilled cooks in the Edible kitchen. Their classmates, the volunteers, and even the teachers, will say, "Oh my gosh, he has completely and finely chopped all that parsley," and then everyone learns a lesson in knife skills and the child's background and life experiences are seen as valuable and cool in a whole different way.

Not only do they interact differently with one another, but their relationships with their teachers change as well. The students begin to see their teachers as people, not just authority figures or sources of necessary yet unwanted information. They become real people who are afraid of bees or aren't good with a pair of pruning shears. They also get the chance to see their teachers learn—often from the students themselves. One story Chapman shared was about a pair of Ethiopian sisters who had recently relocated to the United States. Out in the garden they saw the Edible staff struggling to thresh some grain. When they were able to show them a technique they'd learned in their country of origin, their skills were validated at a time when they really needed it.

Esther Cook, the chef/teacher in the Edible Schoolyard kitchen, was in her ninth year at King Middle School when we spoke with her. She told us that in the beginning she was "completely petrified" by the prospect of having to get kids excited about the vegetables that were coming out of the garden. But over time and while interacting with the students, she eventually came to realize that when kids are happy and enjoying what they're doing, the learning is easy and the food tastes good. What Esther found most remarkable about working with children was how creative they are around food and cooking. She said they have "a natural sense of creativity and beauty." They love to cook. They're happy to be cutting and chopping, mixing and whisking. She doesn't believe in cutting corners—there are no time-saving appliances in her kitchen. Esther believes it's about the whole experience, not just the end product.

The Edible Schoolyard program culminates with the eighth grade *Iron Chef*. Like the chefs on the popular television show, these students use their creativity, communication skills, and teamwork to make a meal from a mystery basket of raw ingredients. For the students who have been at King for three years, it's an opportunity to showcase what they've learned. The results are always interesting and often delicious. For one Iron Chef, the students were given some cooked dried beans, raw beets, radishes, asparagus, oranges, apples, and cheese. They were also allowed to use oil, vinegar, salt, and pepper. If they wanted other spices they had to ask. With forty-five minutes to brainstorm and forty-five minutes to create one hot and one cold dish, the kids had to focus on timing.

Cook described what the teams did with the ingredients they'd been given:

> With the black beans some kids made a dip. Some actually made a chili—they put in some apple, black beans, asked for spices and got cloves and cinnamon and they added radishes and lemon zest, then hollowed out a loaf of bread, put the chili in it, and put the top back on.
>
> Some sautéed the asparagus, others steamed it, and still others broiled it and made a vinaigrette for it. One group made a fruit salad. They were all kind of thrown by the beets, but one girl diligently peeled them and cut them up really tiny and used

A transcontinental head of lettuce grown in California and shipped nearly 3,000 miles to Washington, D.C., requires nearly thirty-six as much fossil fuel energy in transport as it provides in food energy when eaten.

some lemon zest and orange zest and mixed them in with their apples and oranges and it was delicious.

Another group made bruschetta with asparagus on top. Some kids hollowed out the apples and squeezed orange juice and served it in an apple cup. They're phenomenal. You can't imagine the ideas they're going to come up with.

Listening to the brainstorming is incredibly revealing; it's amazing what some of the kids know. One girl today begged me for an egg. "Please can we have an egg, we really want to make an aioli to go over our asparagus." No egg. They made vinaigrette instead.

The children are judged on originality of ideas, hospitality, the flavor of the food, cooperation, and cleanliness. Judges visit each table and talk with the kids about their food, and then have a rigorous judging. Cook said, "The kids are really into this whole competition thing. They want to know whose food was best. They really do want to know and they remember."

Having sensory experiences like cooking and gardening built into their school day really changes kids' fundamental approach to school. It allows them to be themselves, and it opens them up to themselves in ways that never would have happened without this innovative—and in our opinion, essential—approach to education.

Alice Waters truly is the mother of invention when it comes to changing how we feed and educate our children. Her passion and dedication broke new ground, literally, with The Edible Schoolyard over a decade ago, and today those are the very qualities that are making the School Lunch Initiative a reality. Alice believes food and nutrition should become part of the core curriculum. Her philosophy and approach to education are not necessarily embraced by all in the educational community, but Alice won't be swayed. Her vision is to literally teach lunch.

In an interview, she told us about how she envisions the future of school lunch and the school lunch curriculum. "Maybe it's a history class in which the kids are learning about the Middle East and we serve food from the Middle East. We could be talking about it around the table. Or perhaps it's a language class and the students are involved in serving and menu construction and everything is in Spanish and we're serving Mexican food. I think we see lunch as a time to have an interactive experience. It's sort of a lab—the cafeteria is a laboratory, like in a science class."

Lack of funding for innovative programs like the one Alice describes is always presented as a primary problem. Alice believes that we should approach making changes in the school lunch program similarly to the way we changed public school physical fitness programs. We had a president's council on physical fitness, gyms were built, and money was allocated to physical education teachers, sports programs, and physical fitness curriculum. The same can be done with food and nutrition. A president's council would oversee the program, new cafeterias and lunchrooms would be built, and money would be allocated to food-and-nutrition instructors, kitchen-garden programs, and food-and-nutrition curriculum. Alice believes a set of programs like those established for physical fitness are necessary if we are to change how we feed our children and teach them how to eat in ways that benefit their long-term health.

Michele Lawrence, superintendent of the Berkeley Unified School District, explained that throughout the history of public education, lunch hasn't always been the responsibility of school administrators. How we feed children hasn't been considered part of the educational system, but rather it is simply a necessary service provided that just

Pillsbury and General Mills worked with food writers and women's magazines after World War II to convince American housewives that cooking meals from scratch was arduous, old-fashioned, unhygienic, expensive, and generally inferior to prepackaged cake mixes, TV dinners, and frozen scrambled eggs.

kind of "fills in the middle of the day."

After more than thirty years of supervising children while eating her own sandwich on autopilot, it hit Lawrence that school administrators had handed more than thirty to forty-five minutes in the middle of the school day as if it weren't quality time that could be a valuable part of the educational experience. Her vision of the School Lunch Initiative combines changing school food, addressing the ways in which healthful food can be used to combat childhood diseases, and finding a way to use those thirty to forty-five minutes more productively.

Lawrence told us that many school districts are severely underfunded and said,

> It is surprising to me, and has been all my career, that our parents so value their children that they do in-depth research just to buy the safest cars and they spend an enormous amount of time choosing the perfect college or attending to the kind of clothing their children wear. They want very much to make sure they are protected and safe. And then they send them off for the greater portion of their day to public school, which is assigned one of the lesser priorities in our country. They think nothing of buying a ticket for their kid to go to a basketball game that costs $30 or $40 for a single event for a few hours and have no idea that the entire school day for their children in many instances costs less than $25 per day. For six hours.

Indeed, in many schools our tax dollars are paying approximately $4 per hour for our children's education. This includes everything—teachers, chalkboards, libraries, computers, sports, and food—everything. Unbelievable, considering the fact that current average babysitting rates run between $7 and $10 an hour.

What can we do to change this? One answer surely is to get involved. Through legislation we taxpayers can demand that more money be spent on education and on creating healthy school menus. We can also start thinking more creatively. For instance, superintendent

Organic Pop Tarts?

We have been writing together for many years and have grown to respect each other tremendously. Most often we think very alike, however we agree to disagree ever so slightly on organic junk/processed food.

AC: My initial exposure to Chefs Collaborative was at a symposium in Puerto Rico in 1996. On the very first day I found myself sitting under a tent listening to Joan Gussow talk about the growing trend toward organics and the USDA's forthcoming Organic Standards Act. One of the most powerful moments for me was when, as part of her speech, she asked whether "organic food should simply mirror the existing food system, with its highly processed sugary junk food; or should it be something more? Should it also reflect the socially responsible farming practices that were traditionally part of organic and family farming?"

A decade later, I feel strongly that organic junk food is antithetical to healthy food. Every year I go to the Natural Foods Expo and see aisle after aisle after aisle of organic candy, organic fat- and salt-laden chips, organic sugar-coated cereals—and I'm appalled. We need to be teaching our children about healthy food choices—we just don't need an organic Twinkie. We don't!

Sure, I can understand that if McDonald's only served organic french fries all the potatoes in this country would be grown without chemicals, and that would be a good thing. But just because a Twinkie or a gummy bear or an M&M can be organic, doesn't mean that we should promote them to our children. Junk food is junk food—organic or not!

LH: Of course, I agree with her on a very fundamental level. Junk food is junk food and why bother to make it organic? But I tend to think there are varying degrees of junk food and I also believe that not all processed food is junk. As the busy mother of two children I like to know that I can offer them an organic alternative to some of the conventionally processed snack foods that take up so much aisle space in the grocery store. Sometimes kids like to have a treat and maybe the best we can do with the limited time we have is a processed organic cookie. Personally, I'd rather know there are organic choices out there for my kids than not.

Fig Newmans over Fig Newtons? You bet. I work, take care of two kids, run a household, and participate in a host of community activities. I don't have time to bake fig bars every day, and to be honest, it's not even possible for me to procure all the organic ingredients I'd need in order to bake the equivalent here in my own home.

I was faced with a similar situation when I started thinking about my son's and daughter's first foods. I wanted to make my own, but then I realized that there was no way I'd find organic blueberries and winter squash and pears and zucchini in my local market. There may have been a few organic produce items available, but if I stuck with those my children wouldn't have been able to get the variety that is so important to developing bodies and palates. Because I preferred knowing that my kids were getting 100 percent organic food, I opted to buy Earth's Best baby food and recommended it to everyone I know.

Have I fallen into the organic sugared cereal trap? I will sheepishly admit here that yes, I absolutely have because I was in a hurry and being tortured by a four-year-old who wouldn't stop hopping on one leg while begging for a particular sugar-coated chocolate puffed rice cereal. I bought it, we tasted it, and we both came to the conclusion that it was disgusting (while my husband needled me in the background over having paid more for a box of organic junk as opposed to regular junk) and we threw it out. And I learned my lesson.

Just as with everything else in life, it makes little sense to condemn the entire organic processed foods industry because some of what's out there is junk. It's up to us, as parents, to determine which products are good and which aren't. There are some merits to a great many of the processed products we're seeing out there. I'm all for embracing the ones that make sense for my family and, as Ann pointed out, organic on a larger scale is better for the planet anyway.

Lawrence suggested that in California, if 50 cents were added to every entertainment ticket sold, the resulting revenues would solve the state's educational woes. It seems like a small price to pay to solve such an enormous crisis.

Challenges

Each school and school district has its own unique hurdles to cross before implementing the perfect school lunch program, but there are a few system-wide challenges that we have encountered time and time again that must be addressed on a national level by the government, among them: Food preparation and distribution in large-scale school districts like New York, Chicago, and Los Angeles; funding; training; and upgraded facilities.

Food Processing

Karen Wadsworth, a former FoodChange staffer, was the senior program officer of Educational Initiative in the New York City school district. Her main areas of focus were curriculum development (CookShop was on her agenda at the time) and acting as a liaison between two Kellogg Foundation–funded grants: S.O.U.L. Food and SchoolFood Plus—both of which have been increasing the amount of regionally grown agricultural products into institutional kitchens—and the Office of School Food.

Wadsworth had spent a great deal of time working with the Department of Agriculture, farmers' markets, and the Office of School Food to determine the capacity of regional farmers for supplying significant amounts of food to the New York City school kitchens. She serves on the New York State Farm-to-School committee and is a board member at New York Farms, so she has a decided interest in local and sustainable agriculture.

The purpose of CookShop and the SchoolFood Plus Initiative, as we've mentioned, is to increase elementary schoolchildren's consump-

French fries account for 46 percent of vegetable servings eaten by children between the ages of 2 and 19.

tion of whole and minimally processed produce. At the same time, Wadsworth had to balance that noble intention with the school's actual, utterly enormous needs. Her colleague Jennifer Wilkens, a Kellogg food and society policy fellow and Cornell University Farm to School program director, told us that the "issue of scale in agriculture and processing is really coming up as our farm-to-school effort grows in New York. I think when we first started these programs we were looking at one school or one district coming into some association with a limited number of small, but diversified farms . . . but now we're really looking at what structure and what sort of scale is going to work in terms of doing a more localized farm-to-school effort." The processes that worked for Ann in her supply chain at the Ross School, and concepts like The Edible Schoolyard, won't necessarily apply in an urban setting where they're serving nearly a million children a day.

Wadsworth, Wilkens, and the New York City Department of Education's Executive Chef, Jorge Collazo, are making efforts to address the issue of feeding that many children. One of the things that keeps coming up is processing. The goal, both of the Kellogg-funded programs and in school lunch programs generally, is to provide children with as much unprocessed and/or minimally processed food as possible. One of the items the various teams in New York have already successfully used in some schools is a healthy cookie with locally grown butternut squash as its base. If the school district wants to supply all the children in New York City with a cookie made from regionally grown squash, it will have to be prepared at a centralized location and processed to a certain degree. Wilkens said, "As we go in the direction of producing some value-added products on a large scale, we're looking to differentiate it from the kinds of [processed] foods we currently have. . . . Clearly the distances would be less in terms of how far food is being shipped and we will know where things are being grown in the state, so that distinction is very positive. However, since we do have seasons here in New York we will have the issue of needing some value-added processing for the preservation of food." Wilkens went on to talk about the cookie: "It's used as a dessert, but because it has butternut squash in it it can satisfy—depending on the size of the cookie the schools order—either part of or a full vegetable meal component. Basically it's a healthy cookie . . . I'll admit, I was skeptical at first, but I've seen the ingredients list and it's good. It doesn't have a lot of sugar or fat [and uses eggs, squash and honey]; the kids like it." We understand that it's necessary to process some things for a school system as large as New York City's. It just isn't practical to try and bake 3.2 million cookies in the schools. We asked Wilkens how it's possible to take natural, organic, and/or local products and process them without creating yet another heavily processed food for these kids to eat. She admits that this is one of the major questions that has yet to be answered, and there's some tension around it. She looks at it as an

opportunity to rebuild the food system with a diversity in food processing that currently doesn't exist. Because of the nature of school food preparation they need almost everything handled or processed in some way, whether it's a fresh product or something highly processed, so it's an opportunity that this presents for smaller scale, more diversified, more distributed food processing throughout the state. And it may even be that the schools themselves can actually become the centers for this sort of preservation and processing because in many cases they have the infrastructure there. It's also an opportunity for farmers to be engaged in developing some value-added products, either collaboratively or on their own.

As an example, Wilkens cites some work she did with a local potato processor and producer that led to his involvement in school food. He now provides potatoes in several forms (whole, sliced, sliced frozen, cubed, and cubed frozen). That kind of processing is minimal but necessary for schools that have so many mouths to feed every day. Labor costs would simply be too high if all the schools were peeling and cutting their own potatoes every day.

Chef Collazo faces a balancing act between food processing and

Orange juice, bananas, apple juice, apples, grapes, and watermelon make up half of all fruit servings in the United States.

good nutrition every day in his work. He's got a lot of kids to feed and he has to make the right choices for school budgets, food-service workers, and children alike. His department, Culinary Concepts, is successfully establishing new culinary standards for the school system through work with legislators, product design, field testing, and marketing, among other things. Collazo, like the others featured in this chapter, is dedicated to providing kids with high-quality, nutritious foods. Because he is working on such an enormous project, he provides each of the 1,200 schools with field guides to help food-service workers replicate menus and environments system-wide. He was pleasantly surprised to find that the kitchen staff were not only receptive to his initial efforts toward change, but they were also excited about having a chef on board. "They really did care about the kids. I was shocked by the incredible positive energy I felt from these people. They were dedicated and worked very hard, which kind of sealed the deal for me—I knew then that it could work, that we could make great changes."

One of his first projects after taking the job in the spring of 2004 was to create a salad bar field guide. It included designs, recipes, and pictures, and what he found out after the salad bars were in place was that kids actually like salad. Collazo said, "When it's attractive-looking, colorful, clean, and neat, like any other customer, a student will look at it and say, 'Hey, I'd like to have some of that.'" Collazo also makes an effort to bring in processed products that are healthy and have good brand-name appeal—like the Gardenburger he had introduced the day before we interviewed him for this book. He was buoyed by the enthusiasm surrounding that product and told us that he was also starting to add unflavored meats, chicken, and tofu products to school menus. Before he took over, everything was pre-sauced or glazed. "Tofu," he said, "isn't the easiest sell in the world, but if you spice it right and serve it with rice and some meat it moves pretty well." Collazo said he'd like to "move forward with manufacturers, to make the products denser nutritionally," so

Penny-wise and Pound Foolish

When making major changes to improve school food, such as moving from a thaw-and-serve style of food service to cooking from scratch with fresh ingredients, we need to realize how much we're asking of food-service personnel. Every bit of change any of us makes in our lives—when we move, when we change jobs or relationships—is hard.

Revamping school food services requires large changes from a whole group of people, many of whom have been doing their jobs for decades, and have received awards, accolades, and promotions for what they've done. Now we're asking them to unlearn much of what they've learned about preparing school food. We're telling them that they need to acquire new skills, and sometimes to work differently.

Changing the food service will make more sense to workers if they can see themselves as part of a bigger cultural change around food in general, and school food in particular. Historically, the USDA National School Lunch Program has always been treated as a hunger-relief (and farm-support) strategy aimed at undernourished kids. Its success has been measured in pounds of food and numbers of bodies served—never quality, just quantity. The measurements have been calibrated for "How cheap? How many? How much?" In the current crisis of escalating diet-related illnesses, we're living with the consequences of high fat, low-quality food going to increasingly large bodies.

Many food-service employees, especially if they've been doing it for twenty or thirty years, got into school food service because it was a daytime job they could hold while their kids were in school. Over time, many stayed when they discovered that they had a real affinity for feeding kids. Still, most of them are aware of, and uncomfortable with, the fact that the food isn't very good, and the kids don't really appreciate it.

A powerful factor in building enthusiasm for change is remembering that everybody wants to be appreciated for what they do. In many lunchrooms, the lunch ladies are placed in a no-win position. They know that the food isn't good, but they don't have the tools to do anything about it. Being recognized as important players who are improving the school lunch program is tangible, and makes them feel valued and appreciated. When that is the end result, we usually have total buy-in.

I've seen tremendous positive changes in food-service staff when we've improved the food served to students. In one district where I worked, the primary obstacle to change was resistance from the lunch lady in charge. At first, she wanted nothing to do with me and my bunch of young cooks, coming in with our own ideas about how to improve school meals. After we had worked together for about two months, the superintendent called me into his office. "Guess what she served for dinner last night?" he asked. "Roasted vegetables. She brought the leftovers in for me to taste. She said the kids love the food so much, she thought she'd start cooking it at home." Years later, that same lunch lady says that her life changed when the kids she cooked for really began to enjoy the food.

It's also important for people to see the whole picture of what we're trying to change. I don't think that every food-service person has to visit a farm, but every one I've worked with so far has had that opportunity. If you can't get to farms, you should get everyone to a farmers' market. If you can't get to farms or a farmers' market, you need to invite farmers to come to school with an array of freshly harvested food.

If we hope to improve school meals, we've got to begin to measure success in a very different way. In order to do that, we need to begin to think in a very different way. We've got to stop counting pennies, pounds, and people. The issue is not about spending less—or even about spending more. We need a different worldview based on measuring the health of children and the health of the planet. That will lead us to the health of families, communities, farms, and the environment.

The Centers for Disease Control and Prevention recently predicted that 30 to 40 percent of all the kids born in the United States are going to have diabetes in their lifetimes. The percentage is even higher for Hispanic and African American children. We need to ask, "What does that cost?" We currently spend $115 billion on diet-related illness every year, and that number can be expected to grow exponentially. Can we take some of that money and put it into preventative medicine? And can we begin to see healthy school meals and sustainable farming practices as preventative medicine? We need to measure success not by how little of this or how much of that, but by what is good in the long run for children and the planet. Whatever that costs in the near term, we all need to start figuring out how to fund it.

This essay, written by Ann Cooper, is part of Thinking Outside the Lunchbox, an ongoing series of essays connected to the Center for Ecoliteracy's Rethinking School Lunch program. Read all the essays at www.ecoliteracy.org.

Both take-out and restaurant food tend to be higher in fat and calories than food prepared at home.

---

he works closely with manufacturers as he seeks alternative ingredients like Ultragrain, which is 100 percent whole wheat, but is white in color. "The more I start to learn about what's happening in the world of technology and food, those are the types of things I hope to bring to the students and the food. It will be seamless to them, they won't even see it, but it all adds up to a better-looking product, a better-tasting product, a product with better texture." This statement seems utterly contrary to what we've just spent the better part of this book promoting, but in this setting it does have its merits. For one thing, school lunch participation is up in the high schools, which is remarkable given all the choices these kids have in the blocks surrounding their schools. Breakfast participation continues to rise as well. For now, for this enormous school district, it's the way to go—at least until we find a way to provide children in urban schools with the same types of foods and food services that are available to children in smaller school districts around the country.

What? Schools Don't Have Kitchens?

Even if schools get the whole, unprocessed foods we want them to have, there's still a major hurdle to cross. As we see it, the biggest challenges lie in the infrastructure. For starters, school kitchens are severely lacking in equipment. In some cases kitchens are virtually nonexistent. In Berkeley, which is typical of many districts, some kitchens have nothing but "hot boxes" to heat and hold premade processed food. In some kitchens we have been in, we've seen a refrigerator, a freezer, a sink, and then nothing else but these hot-boxes. Of course, there are some fully equipped school kitchens, but they are certainly not the norm. Staff workers are undertrained because as our reliance on processed food has grown we have stopped cooking in schools. Currently kitchen staff workers don't need to know the first thing about cooking. That has to change.

How can we fix this? First and foremost we need to make an investment in our schools to regain the cooking kitchens we've lost over the years. Beyond that we have to hire food-service workers who know how to cook. It's imperative that we pay them a fair wage and offer them health benefits. As an alternative, cooking could also be done in central kitchens, and satellite school kitchens would finish and serve the food.

We also need to spend more money on food. The current average reimbursement rate is $2.34 for a "free" school lunch, with the reimbursement funds coming from the USDA—from our tax dollars. Of this $2.34, typically on average only 80 to 90 cents is spent on the food; the rest is used to cover payroll and overhead. That figure includes the cost of milk and fruit, both National School Lunch Program requirements. Milk costs approximately 18 to 20 cents per lunch. With the remaining 50 to 60 cents, school districts are expected to serve children a nutritious, flavorful 600- or 700-calorie lunch. Can you do that in your kitchen at home? Could you even go to the grocery store and find something with around 700 healthy calories that costs 60 cents? We're chefs and we can't figure out a way to do that. It's no wonder the school districts can't. No one has ever run an economic model to discover the positive impact we could have on school lunch if we added another 50 cents, as in the case of Appleton Central Alternative School, or even a dollar. We need to understand how much money it takes to guarantee a healthy, nutritious lunch that encourages good eating habits for our children.

Beyond all that, we have to reinforce and support all the changes we're making to school lunch programs by educating the children about good nutrition.

In 1992, the USDA conducted a study called the School Nutrition Dietary Assessment. The study found that none of the school lunches at that time were meeting the USDA's own dietary guidelines. In fact,

A recent study showed that teenagers served a fast-food lunch ate an average of 1652 calories during the single meal—more than 60 percent of their estimated daily energy requirement.

they were nearly 50 percent higher in fat than they should have been. School food wasn't about nutrition; it was a business in which the bottom line took precedence over the health of the children being fed. Results of studies conducted around that time at Cornell University indicated that children's eating habits are formed by the time they are twelve years old. The USDA's School Meals Initiative, finalized in 1995, was intended to set guidelines for schools—and, by extension, children—for healthy eating. Not all schools followed the School Meals Initiative to the letter, and using loopholes, a large number of them began installing vending machines and contracting with fast-food companies to increase revenues. It didn't matter what was on the school lunch menu because kids could get junk food at every turn. And they were none the wiser because nutrition education programs fell short. Either they weren't a mandatory part of the curriculum or the school district chose not to participate at all.

Kids who were 5 years old when the School Meals Initiative was put in place in 1995 are 15 years old now. They've passed that critical mark discovered by the researchers at Cornell. They've grown up in a school lunch program that has been faulty at best. Statistics indicating diet-related poor health in children continue to rise. Ellen Haas, CEO of FoodFit and former undersecretary for food, nutrition, and consumer services at the USDA, believes that one way to combat the disconnect between the national and state agencies is to appoint someone to a leadership role "to get people moving, to get things changed. It could be a secretary, an undersecretary, a food-service director, the president of ASFSA, or even state child nutrition directors. The USDA sets them up and sets the enforcement but it's really up to the local level, not up to the Department of Agriculture, to execute and implement them."

Marion Nestle, author of *Food Politics* and chair of New York University's Department of Nutrition, Food Studies, and Public Health, believes that

> We have to hire people who really care. And I mean that really seriously, because if you don't have people who really care in place it's just not going to happen no matter what you do. You can have the best ingredients in the world and if people don't want to play with them or the parents object or the principal just isn't interested, you're just not going to have anything . . . [On top of that] a significant amount of reeducation has got to take place, among the kids. Kids have to understand that this isn't something that is being done to them, that this is an opportunity and it is something that is exciting and innovative and different. In places where this has worked, there's a completely different attitude about different food than in places where people just don't care about what their kids are eating. It's really dramatic to see [the difference]. It requires involving parents in what's going on and it requires a good deal of backup classroom instruction. It also requires hands-on dealing with kids around food issues, and not very many schools have personnel to do this.

Get in Line at the Virtual Cafeteria Online

These days, kids in Texas's Carrollton-Farmers Branch Independent School District can get some of their lunch lessons online when they load their trays with items from the "virtual cafeteria." The animated simulation of school lunch choices is complete with a lunch lady who offers kudos for kids who make healthy food choices. We think it's a great tool that parents can use to teach their children how to eat better with the options available to them at their schools.

Carrollton-Farmers Branch Independent School District, "The Virtual Cafeteria," accessed at http://studentnutrition.cfbisd.edu (click on "Virtual Cafeteria")

When the people who are involved in successful school lunch programs like Appleton and Martin Luther King Middle School talk about the positive changes they've made, their enthusiasm is contagious. Beth Collins, executive chef at the Ross School, was right when she told us that to overcome the challenges inherent in the public school setting someone needs to "create a spark of enthusiasm . . . on every level of the operation from the superintendent to the school board to the parents, the students, the managers in the kitchens." It's our job as parents and educators to initiate that spark.

What Can Parents and Caregivers Do?

First and foremost, we have to stop relying on the government to do the right thing for our kids. As Marion Nestle points out, "It's all a matter of politics and will, and if there was a real national concern about doing something, something would get done. In the meantime parents are going to have to do it on the grassroots level."

We agree with Nestle, even today as nationally mandated, school-district wellness committees have been formed around the country and are looking toward developing wellness policies that will charge local school districts with setting targets for nutrition education and physical activity as well as standards for all foods sold in school, including items sold à la carte, in school stores, and even in vending machines. Senator Tom Harkin (D-IA) said in his speech at the Healthy Schools Summit in Washington, D.C., that "these local wellness policies could be the real sleeper success story of 2004's child nutrition reauthorization. Local wellness policies have the potential to transform the way schools promote child health." When you read this the new policies will be in place in your local school district, but there is still much work to be done.

A bottle of Coke in 1916 held 6.5 ounces; today a regular can of Coke holds 12 ounces; 20-ounce bottles are the vending machine standard; and 32-ounce bottles are widely sold.

Wellness policies will not necessarily be properly implemented just because they exist. We've seen government-mandated programs fall by the wayside where the NSLP is concerned before, and it's much too soon to tell what these new wellness policies will accomplish. It will be up to parents to stay in touch with their school administrators and form committees that monitor school menus, fitness programs, and even the nutrition curriculum if there is one. Concerned parents can start newsletters to keep other parents involved and informed, and may even choose to use the Internet to disburse information through a wellness policy website created for their school or school district or a less formal blog or bulletin board. Most important of all, parents need to maintain a dialogue with their children on this issue to see how effective the new policy programs are.

The reauthorization act wasn't especially clear about how these policies should be implemented, either. In November 2005, Ann was invited to speak to the Wellness Policy Committee of the Napa Valley Unified School District. It was their third meeting, and Ann was giving a speech to reinforce why this work is so important. In attendance were more than thirty members of the community including school administrators, parents, teachers, and students. They were all there because they care about what the schools are feeding children. After Ann spoke, the question-and-answer period was lively:

How do we implement the policies?
Who pays for the changes?
How do we educate both the parents and the students?
How do we change the food service companies and their employees?

Over and over again operational questions like these come up. The truth is we're really going to have to take a wait-and-see attitude about that part of it. What we do know is that the very call for wellness policies is a positive and hopeful step. How successful they are will ultimately still depend on parents and administrators. What we are hoping is that good, strong policies will be in place in June 2006, and that they will take a multiyear approach to the adjustments that need to be made so that changes will be made slowly yet constantly, until every school reaches even their highest goal.

Nothing should be written in stone. There should be ongoing plans that include social marketing to—and the education of—all of the stakeholders including parents, students, school administrators, and food-service workers. Since there is no money in the law for enforcement, parents and caregivers need to be part of the solution by making sure that individual schools and school districts maintain ongoing food-policy committees that continually "check in" on the food. There should also be a reporting structure in place that will allow for constant improvements to the policies and programs themselves, and the policies should be updated annually. Make your voice count: Let it be heard over and over and over again.

In his speech to the Healthy Schools Summit, Harkin went on to say that

> the onus should not be entirely on local people. We need a more active federal government in setting guidance for public schools. To that end, I am sponsoring the Child Nutrition Promotion and School Lunch Protection Act of 2005. Among other things, this bill would update nutrition standards for all foods sold in schools. Currently, under thirty-year-old USDA standards, it's just fine for schools to sell ice cream, Oreos, Snickers candy bars, donuts, and all kinds of other junk foods. Obviously, it's time to update USDA standards based on all that we have learned about nutrition and obesity over the last three decades.
>
> In addition, my bill would close the giant loophole that

In a large, federally funded study, researchers found that a diet containing 8 to 10 servings of fruits and vegetables per day effectively reduced blood pressure.

says: USDA can set standards for foods sold in the lunchroom, but cannot set standards for foods sold elsewhere on campus, including right outside the cafeteria. This loophole is a disaster. It means USDA spends nearly $9 billion a year on nutritious breakfasts and lunches, but this is undermined—sabotaged is a better word—by the pervasive sale of junk food and sugary sodas elsewhere on campus. That's a loophole you can drive a Pepsi delivery truck through—and we need to close it!

Parents have to support and expand upon what kids will be learning in school. You can start by not buying things you don't want your kids to eat. It may sound easy, but it's not. Marion Nestle told us that she's

> very sympathetic to parents about what they go through with food. Their kids are being subjected to [billions of dollars] a year worth of marketing directed specifically at 8- to 12-year-olds. [The marketing] does three things. It establishes brand loyalty, encourages kids to pester their parents (just watch one ad and you'll know where that comes from), and it is designed to convince kids that they need their own special kind of food. Once you understand that this is marketing that is designed to undermine parental controls, it loses that "isn't-that-cute" factor. It isn't cute at all, it's quite subversive.

In buying this book you've taken the first step toward shutting down the marketing machine that threatens your children's health. You've made a commitment to rescue them from a lifetime of poor diet and nutrition. Preparing healthful lunches with whole ingredients will make a tremendous difference in the way they play and learn. Teaching them about good nutrition combined with physical activity will give them the tools they need to maintain good future health. Getting involved in school food wellness programs will change the lives of an entire generation of children for the better. Now is the time to get involved. Just do it. Just do one thing: You can make a difference.

> No nation is any healthier than
> its children—the well nourished
> school child is a better student.
> He is healthier and more alert.
> He is developing good food
> habits that will benefit him for
> the rest of his life. In short, he is
> a better asset for his country in
> every way.
>
> —HARRY TRUMAN

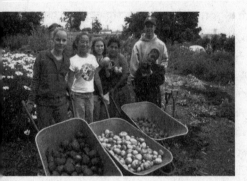

CHAPTER 3

Beyond the Lunch Pail

Good health extends well beyond good nutrition. There are all sorts of things can you do to make your child's world a richer, healthier place. You can eliminate potential health hazards, including cleaning and gardening products; you can bring gardening and composting into your family's daily life; and you can use your buying power to support businesses that provide you with local, organic, and sustainable healthy food choices.

Before we begin, it is important to note that while researching the potential danger of household products we found that there is all manner

King Middle School children harvesting potatoes *The Chez Panisse Foundation*

Research shows that 80 percent of all cancer can be prevented through healthful diet and exercise.

of conflicting information, especially online. The incredible benefit we all share in using the Internet can also be confusing and cause us to go into absolute information overload. In exactly whom and what should we believe?

We've decided, when making suggestions that will potentially affect the long-term health and well-being of our children, to invoke the Precautionary Principle, which, at its core, admonishes us, as our mothers did, that it is better to be safe than sorry. Or, further, that "when an activity raises threats of harm to human health or the environment, precautionary measures should be taken even if some cause-and-effect relationships are not fully established scientifically." (from the January 1998 *Wingspread Statement on the Precautionary Principle*).

If, as a result of our research, we believe that there is a modicum of potential harm in a practice, technology, or product—even if the research is refuted—we will suggest steering clear of it. None of us wants to roll the dice on something that has the potential, however small, to cause our children harm, particularly because pound for pound their exposure to potentially harmful products is often higher.

Live Green!

The Earth does not belong to us. As we've often heard said, we hold it in trust for and borrow it from our children. Take that to heart and make a commitment to pay back the loan with interest. For the sake of our children we ought to be working toward leaving the Earth in better shape than we found it. Implement these simple steps and you'll be well on your way.

🐟 REDUCE WASTE. Don't let a little wear and tear send you off on a shopping spree. Make repairs to damaged goods and increase their longevity. Avoid excess packaging—a large percentage of our municipal solid waste stream is the result of unnecessary packaging. When given a choice, select the product that is most sensibly packaged.

꙳ REUSE. Compost kitchen scraps (for more info see page 111), pack lunches in reusable bags and lunch boxes, use reusable water bottles, and choose unbleached organic cotton diapers over disposables. Diaper production alone consumes more than 80,000 pounds of plastic and 200,000 trees a year in the United States. Filling the landfills with so much waste threatens our access to clean water by polluting rivers and streams. Numerous companies, including Eco-Products, carry compostable trash and leaf bags. Biodegradable shopping bags also help reduce landfill waste, so ask your local supermarkets to use them. Better yet, purchase some reusable canvas tote bags to use instead of the plastic or paper bags. Keep them in the trunk of your car so you'll have them on hand when you do your shopping.

꙳ RECYCLE. Recycle everything you can. Cans and bottles are the easy stuff, but with a little extra effort there are other things in your house that you can recycle: computers, household hazardous waste, motor oil, cardboard, paper, and even phone books. For comprehensive information on how and where to recycle in your area visit www.earth911.org and search using your ZIP code. Support recycling by making a special effort to buy recycled products. While recycling is the first step, the recycling loop isn't complete until the materials collected curbside and at drop-off sites are remanufactured into new products and purchased by consumers. The fewer virgin resources that go into products, the better.

꙳ BE EFFICIENT. Whether it's a car or a computer, choose the most energy-efficient model. For electrical appliances, look for the Energy Star logo. Conventional lightbulbs (incandescent) use significantly more energy than compact fluorescents, which not only last ten times longer, but produce half the carbon dioxide in their lifetime. Batteries, which power most of today's kids' toys—not to mention

---

35 percent of American children are overweight—25 percent of those are obese and 12 percent have type 2 diabetes.

⤼| 1 out of every 4 meals in our country is eaten in a fast-food outlet.

handheld video games and MP3 players—contain dangerous toxins that should be treated as hazardous waste. We use and throw away millions of them every year. Rechargeable batteries cost more at first, but once you have a good system of use going you'll not only be protecting the earth, you'll be saving money. Transportation and fossil fuels are currently at the forefront of the national consciousness because gas prices have skyrocketed. If you're not already car-pooling kids and have a big enough car to fit a few more car seats, start now. Take public transportation if it's available, and dust off your old bicycle. Most recently, hybrid cars have made an appearance and have become so popular that in some places waiting lists are more than six months long. Independently of each other we both bought Toyota Priuses this year and love them. It's hard to understand why anyone would want to drive anything else, frankly. At 45 to 55 miles per gallon, these cars are a much less expensive ride and the technology is just too incredible to ignore.

🖎 READ LABELS. Whenever possible, look for labels that let you know the product is certified as environmentally friendly. But be careful—don't blindly accept a product that calls itself "green" but doesn't offer any substantiation. To get smart on what labels mean, visit Consumers Union's Eco-labels website, www.eco-labels.org. Make a point to avoid plastics made from polyvinyl chloride (PVC), labeled #3 plastic. It's a leading source of dioxin (a potent toxin) in the environment.

🖎 BE SMART ABOUT PAPER PRODUCTS. Buy paper with the highest percentage of post-consumer waste, and when possible, choose paper that is process chlorine free. Why? Because 38.9 percent of all waste in the average American home is paper, which is made from materials that contribute to deforestation and global warming, and which most often ends up back in the landfill. Think about all the paper that goes into a typical school year for your child and multiply that by millions and millions of schoolchildren. Buying paper products high in postconsumer recycled content will help alleviate some of the stress on the planet.

Busy parents are often stretched thin. One favorite time-saver, especially in the summer or on weekends, is disposable dinnerware. We will always advocate the use of real dishes, glassware, and silverware, but when that's not practical, we suggest biodegradable and compostable paper goods as an alternative to paper, plastic, and Styrofoam. New technologies have enabled manufactures to utilize sugar cane, potatoes, wheat, and corn to produce disposable-ware that actually composts in one or two weeks. These dishes, cups, and utensils can be thrown right in your compost pile. For more information on those types of products, check out Eco-Products (www.ecoproducts.com). A surprisingly attractive alternative is Forestware (www.eatitworld.com), made from the leaves of tropical plants and fully compostable.

Lunch Boxes and Food Storage

We recommend the Laptop Lunch Box System (p. 160), especially in light of the recent revelation that a great many children's soft vinyl lunch boxes contain lead. In August 2005, the Center for Environmental Health (CEH) filed lawsuits against makers and retailers of soft vinyl lunch boxes because, as Michael Green, executive director of CEH put it, "Lead exposure should not be on the lunch menu when kids go back to school this fall. . . ." Lead is known to cause hyperactivity, irritability, lack of focus, and in the worst cases, damage to overall brain development. CEH asserts that laboratory testing found seventeen lunch boxes with unacceptably high levels of lead. For the most up-to-date information about lead in lunch boxes visit www.cehca.org/html.

85 percent of American children do not sit down to a meal on a regular basis.

The Plastic Polemic

To save resources, it makes sense to pack our children's lunch items in reusable plastic containers. It's convenient and they are easy to clean and store. Cottage cheese, frozen soup, even take-out Chinese food come in plastic containers sturdy enough to wash, save, and reuse. Most can be safely run through the dishwasher and stored with food in the refrigerator.

Trouble is, some research is showing that heating and reusing plastic containers is potentially harmful. There's also research that says it's perfectly safe. This is one instance in which we prefer to invoke the Precautionary Principle and advise you to heat foods in regular dishes whenever possible. Saving those old reuseable containers will be perfectly safe for a short time, but be careful about reusing, refreezing, and remicrowaving plastics, especially those labeled #1 and #3. The chemicals used to make the plastic will eventually begin to break down with exposure to extreme temperatures, and potentially poisonous compounds will leach into the food. We suggest glass and ceramic for storage, reheating, and microwaving.

Plastic wraps may contain dioxins and DEHA (diethylhydroxylamine), both of which are potential carcinogens. There is some evidence that those compounds can migrate onto food when heated, especially greasy, fatty foods. We recommend that you not use plastic wrap to reheat your children's foods in the microwave. Use glass or ceramic dinnerware and cover with a lid made from a like material or a dampened paper towel. If you have no choice but to use plastic wrap when reheating, make sure it doesn't touch the food.

Water

Water is of utmost importance to the body. Generally speaking, you can't drink too much of it. In the 1990s bottled water flooded the mar-

> ✂ Food companies in America are spending more per child on advertising than any other nation in the world, $15 billion per year marketing food to kids, which is more than what it would cost to provide health insurance for all uninsured children.

ketplace. Before we knew it, those clear plastic bottles (with and without sports caps) were everywhere. Virtually overnight it became a multibillion dollar industry. We currently consume more than 4 billion gallons of bottled water each year—so much that soda companies have identified water as a significant and growing part of their business. Much of it is sold to us by Coke and Pepsi, and we spend nearly $10,000 per minute on something that was once considered free. Virtually all of it is packaged in disposable plastic containers, the very same plastic containers that may contain chemicals suspected of leaching into the products they contain. A great deal of that plastic ultimately

Some Key Differences Between EPA Tap Water and FDA Bottled Water Rules						
WATER TYPE	DISINFECTION REQUIRED?	CONFIRMED *E. COLI* & FECAL COLIFORM BANNED?	TESTING FREQUENCY FOR BACTERIA	MUST FILTER TO REMOVE PATHOGENS, OR HAVE STRICTLY PROTECTED SOURCE?	MUST TEST FOR *CRYPTO-SPORIDIUM, GIARDIA,* VIRUSES?	TESTING FREQUENCY FOR MOST SYNTHETIC ORGANIC CHEMICALS
Bottled Water	No	No	1/Week	No	No	1/year
Carbonated or seltzer water	No	No	None	No	No	None
Big city tap water (using surface water)	Yes	Yes	Hundreds/month	Yes	Yes	1/quarter (limited waivers available if clean source)
See Table 1 of NRDC's bottled water report for further comparisons and explanations. http://www.nrdc.org/water/drinking/nbw.asp						

ends up in landfills where, ironically, it may sit, polluting our fresh, clean water supplies for generations to come.

Plastic pollution aside, not many of us give much thought to the water itself. We should be asking ourselves whether bottled water is, in fact, better than tap water. The Natural Resource Defense Council (NRDC) suggests that in many cases, not only is tap water healthier than bottled water, but that it is more highly regulated than bottled water. You may not be surprised to learn that much of our bottled water is just tap water with fancy packaging and high-priced advertising.

One NRDC study tested more than 1,000 bottles of 103 brands of bottled water. While most of the tested waters were found to be of high quality, some brands were contaminated. About one-third of the waters tested contained levels of contamination, including synthetic chemicals, bacteria, and arsenic. One of the key findings in the NRDC study was that bottled water regulations do not adequately protect us and our children. The water, in some cases, is neither pure nor safe.

The Food and Drug Administration is the governing agency whose job it is to protect us from impure and unsafe bottled water. They test for allowable amounts of contaminants (which, incidentally, are higher than the allowable limits in tap water), but their jurisdiction does not extend to water that is bottled and sold in the same state. That accounts for between 60 and 70 percent of all the bottled water sold in the United States. In essence, the majority of our bottled water slips through the cracks in federal oversight. The graph on page 95 gives weight to the NRDC's arguments.

Our thoughts? Bottled water is an expensive, unnecessary part of most of our lives. If you are concerned about the tap water in your area, have it tested and research a filtering system for your drinking water. Choose glass-lined or stainless steel over plastic for water containers. When plastic is your only alternative, choose #2, #4, or #5 plastics (look on the bottom of the bottle inside the recycling sym-

---

Our children watch more than 10,000 food-related commercials every year—most for high-sugar and high-fat foods.

> Food marketing in our country has become big business: In the United States
> we produce 3800 calories for every person and most of us should be eating
> less than two-thirds of that.

bol) because these types have the smallest health and environmental
impacts.

Cleaning Products

When we think about cleaning products, we think about products that
make our job easier and faster. Advertising admonishes us to have
"white," "clean," "sanitary" homes, but often the chemicals that leave
all of our surfaces sparkling may have a hazardous impact on our health
and the health of our children. Some of these chemicals are poisonous,
others can burn skin or eyes (ever walk down a grocery store aisle
overflowing with cleaning products of every scent and variety and got-
ten to the end with burning, watering eyes?) and still others, like chlorine bleach, can wreak havoc on the environment. A few safe, simple
ingredients like soap, water, baking soda, vinegar, lemon juice, and bo-
rax, in combination with a little elbow grease and a coarse sponge for
scrubbing, can take care of most household cleaning needs. They can
also save you lots of money wasted on unnecessary, specialized cleaners.
This is again an area to invoke the Precautionary Principle, when in
doubt, not only err on the side of safety but simplicity as well. Some of
our favorite green cleaning supply companies are: Seventh Generation,
Simple Green, Planet, Ecover, and Earth Friendly Products. We love
Seventh Generation's laundry detergent and Earth Friendly's olive and
orange oil wood furniture polish. And a mixture of 3 parts water to 1 part
white vinegar makes a great, inexpensive all-purpose cleaner.

If you're not sure where to begin we recommend the Green Guide
as a resource. The National Green Pages and the Green Guide Smart
Shoppers Card on page 98 can help you locate the green products that
are best for you and your family.

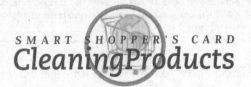

SMART SHOPPER'S CARD

CleaningProducts

from

THEGreenGuide

P.O. Box 567 Prince Street Station, NY, NY 10012
(212) 598-4910 . www.thegreenguide.com

RECOMMENDED HOUSEHOLD CLEANING PRODUCTS

Dishwashing Liquids & Dishwasher Detergents

Trader Joe's Next to Godliness Liquid Dish Soap
Trader Joe's stores - find locations at traderjoes.com; 800-SHOP-TJS

Ecover Natural Dishwashing Liquid
At stores nationwide - ecover.com; 800-449-4925

Seventh Generation Free & Clear Dish Powder (or liquid)
At stores nationwide or online - seventhgeneration.com; 802-658-3773

Earth Friendly Products Dishmate
At stores nationwide or online - ecos.com; 800-335-ECOS

Laundry Products

Seventh Generation Free & Clear Laundry Powder (or liquid)
At stores nationwide or online - seventhgeneration.com; 802-658-3773

Earth Friendly Products Ecos Liquid Laundry Detergent
At stores nationwide or online - ecos.com; 800-335-ECOS

Ecover Natural Laundry Wash Ultra (liquid) & Laundry Powder
At stores nationwide - ecover.com; 800-449-4925

Window Cleaners

Aubrey Organics Liquid Sparkle Spray Cleaner
Available online - aubreyorganics.com; 800-282-7394

Trader Joe's Home E-Zen-tials No-Streak Multipurpose Cleaner
Trader Joe's stores - find locations at traderjoes.com; 800-SHOP-TJS

Scrubs

Bon Ami
At stores nationwide - bonami.com

Earth Friendly Cream Cleanser
At stores nationwide or online - ecos.com; 800-335-ECOS

Floor Cleaners

Murphy Oil Soap
At stores nationwide or online - murphyoilsoap.com

Ecover Floor Soap with Natural Linseed Oil
At stores nationwide - ecover.com; 800-449-4925

Multipurpose Cleaners

Dr. Bronner's Sal Suds
At stores nationwide - drbronner.com; 760-743-2211

Aubrey Organics Earth Aware Household Cleanser
Available online - aubreyorganics.com; 800-282-7394

Vermont Soapworks Organic Liquid Sunshine Nontoxic Cleanser
At stores nationwide or online - vermontsoap.com; 866-762-7482

Toilet Cleaners

Bioshield Toilet Bowl Cleanser
Available online - bioshieldpaint.com; 800-621-2591

Seventh Generation Toilet Bowl Cleaner
At stores nationwide or online - seventhgeneration.com; 802-658-3773

For more information go to www.thegreenguide.com

Dining and Shopping Alternatives

It has been said that eating is a political act and that we vote with our forks, or, essentially, with our food-purchasing dollar. It does make a difference whether we shop at a farmers' market or Wal-Mart, or whether we take our children to eat at a fast-food franchise every night or whether we actually cook at home with them. What follows are a few alternatives to the mainstream mega-store shopping and dining experiences.

We don't have to succumb to the primary fast-food dining choices out there. There are quick-serve casual establishments that are better for our children's health. In the Northeast there is a small chain, O'Naturals, founded by Gary Hirschberg of Stonyfield Yogurt. O'Naturals' mission is summed up by this proclamation on their wall: "Ingredients: We have this crazy idea that your food ought to be 100 percent food. All of our ingredients are free of additives, preservatives, artificial flavors, colors, sweeteners and hydrogenated oils." Another fast-food chain, Chipotle Grill, founded by Steve Ells, believes in "Food With Integrity," which means,

> going back along the food chain . . . going beyond distributors to discover how the vegetables are grown, how the pigs, cows and chickens are raised, where the best spices come from. Take our carnitas, for example. In pursuing new sources of pork, we discovered naturally raised pigs from a select group of farmers. These animals are not confined in stressful "factories." They live outdoors or in deeply bedded pens, so they are free to run, roam, root and socialize. They are not given hormones or antibiotics.

The CDC has stated that of the children born in the year 2000, 30 to 40 percent will contract diabetes.

FullBloom Baking Company: A Truly Socially Responsible Company

While it's great to get your family directly involved in cooking and gardening projects, it's also essential to teach your children how important it is to support local food-related businesses that ameliorate the community through sustainable practices. FullBloom Baking Company is a perfect example of the type of business we see as an essential part of a healthy future for our country.

Karen Trilevsky began FullBloom Baking Company in 1989 in a borrowed kitchen, where she baked all night and napped on flour sacks. The back of her pickup truck served as her makeshift delivery van. Over the course of 16 years the company has grown to more than 200 employees who service more than 500 wholesale accounts out of a 60,000-square-foot baking facility with state-of-the-art equipment. In the food-service business that story alone would be impressive, but Karen's story is bigger than that. Hers is the story of an entrepreneur who has built a business that is the model of sustainability.

FullBloom's employees, most of whom are Hispanic, are all paid a living wage and every one of them has full health benefits, which in the food-service business is a rarity on both counts. If Karen had stopped there she would be giving her employees more than the average food-service employer does, but she also started the Smart Cookie Foundation, which is open to the larger community and supports first-generation immigrant children in their quest to go to college. As of this writing, more than thirty children of FullBloom employees as well as eight employees are succeeding in secondary-level education. As if that isn't amazing enough, Karen also gives back-to-school gift certificates for clothes, books, and supplies to her employees with school-age children and has established an activities fund that allows the children of employees to attend art and activities classes and sports, and gives them access to tutoring if needed. On-site classes include computers, management, English as a Second Language (ESL), first aid, ServeSafe (national food-service sanitation certification), and even yoga!

Her eye toward sustainability isn't just limited to her employees. The FullBloom team strives to make Karen's business a leader in environmental practices as well. Many FullBloom staff have company cars, all of which are Hybrid Priuses; she received organic certification in 2004; and she has implemented extensive recycling policies and through dedication has reduced her waste stream by three-quarters in the past five years.

Karen and her team also give back to their communities by supporting local nonprofit organizations whose missions have meaning to FullBloom's employees. From supporting AIDS research to antidiscrimination policies and immigration activism, FullBloom helps support a wide range of community causes. Most recently, FullBloom embarked on a collaboration with the Berkeley Unified School District that promotes and supports universal breakfast throughout the school district. We believe that this type of public/private partnership is one of the keys to getting better food on our children's plates at school.

FullBloom effectively raises the bar in every way, and proves that it is an intrinsic operating imperative that successful, financially vibrant companies can and do excel when they embrace socially responsible operating policies. The "triple bottom line,"—the harmonious coexistence of employees, the environment, and profit—really can support the growth and success of businesses in the food-service industry. We hope more visionaries like Karen will embrace this sustainable approach to their businesses and work toward building companies that truly make a difference. One way for them to do that is for you, as consumers, to show your support with your purchasing dollars.

While we believe that cooking and eating at home is the healthiest option, we also know that going out to eat can be a fun and worthwhile family event. We just ask that when you do go out, drive by those giant fast-food places and seek out the O'Naturals and Chipotle Grills of your hometown. Vote with your food dollar and patronize restaurants that produce healthier food and support a sustainable food system.

Some of our favorite places to shop are farmers' markets and farm stands. From San Francisco's Ferry Plaza and New York City's Union Square Greenmarket to the tiny one-man-show roadside farm stands of

In less than 200 years we have gone from being a nation of farmers (more than 95 percent) to a nation in which less than 2 percent of the population grows our food.

backwoods towns, they are hands down the best places to get fresh, local produce. The only way you can get closer to the source is to pick the food yourself. Buying direct from farmers is one of the most important ways we can shop. It keeps farmers farming, gets healthy food on your plate, and enables your children to make the connection between the food on their plate and the people who worked so hard to grow it. To find farmers' markets and other local food sources in your area, check out: www.foodroutes.org.

An intermediate step between farmers' markets and supermarkets are food cooperatives (co-ops). In more than 500 communities nationwide, food co-ops are flourishing. Once seen as a haven for hippies, these contemporary employee- or customer-owned businesses are taking the place of mega-stores for many families. In Vermont we have both shopped at the Putney Co-op and the Brattleboro Co-op, both of which feature organic and natural products as well as local seasonal produce. In Brooklyn, New York, the famous Park Slope Co-op, founded in 1973, has become the largest wholly member-owned and operated food co-op in the country with more than 11,000 members. So whether you live in a rural community or one of the largest urban areas in the country, you can seek out food co-ops and buying clubs that will help bring healthier food to your family's plate.

Now, we understand that those shopping options are a sort of utopian ideal. We know how easy it is to shop at the major chain food stores, too—especially with kids in tow. Everything is right there, no need to hop from one store to another dragging kids in and out of car seats in the cold and rain. We realize that not everyone will be able to—or even want to—shop at a farmers' market. Those of us who do, will need to augment our shopping in grocery stores. This is where voting with your dollars makes a huge difference. Wal-Mart is now the largest food purveyor in the world, but there are alternatives. The organic and natural foods industry is growing at a rate of 20 percent a year, which is fueling expansion by chains like Whole Foods. Whole Foods' food isn't necessarily all organic or local, but much of it is and they are highly responsive to questions and requests. Other chains are beginning to habitually stock organic produce and hormone- and antibiotic-free meat and dairy. When shopping in grocery stores, ask questions of the store or department managers. If you don't see the food you'd like to be feeding your children, ask them to get it. The more people make requests for local and organic food, the sooner we'll see more healthy products on grocery store shelves.

Lawn and Garden Care

While it's important to protect your family inside the walls of your home with healthy food and green cleaning products, it's equally important for us to clean up our act right outside our own front doors. The lawn care industry spreads almost 100 million pounds or $2 billion of chemicals onto the lawns, trees, shrubs, and plants of America each year. This statistic is somewhat incredible on its own, but when you realize that figure is ten times more per acre than is typically used on farmland, it's staggering. Many of us are obsessed with bright green picture-perfect lawns, which adorn more than 30 million acres of this country's land. The path to that bright green lawn, for most homeowners, is paved with more than 200 government-approved chemicals. Many of them can make your family ill. Not only is contact with many of these chemicals harmful, but the effect they have on our ground and drinking water can be devastating.

Depending on your level of comfort and dedication, there are many alternatives to chemical lawn care. The Northeastern Organic Farming Association (NOFA) has developed a program and published *Standards*

---

3 percent of farms in the United States produce 47 percent of the crops.

Think Globally, Eat Locally

Brian Halweil

About a year after I joined the staff of Worldwatch, a columnist for the conservative *Washington Times* took advantage of me. During a long interview about what it was like to work at an environmental group, he honed in on one out-of-context statement I had made about how hard it could be to research and write on trends—biodiversity decline, population growth, the spread of AIDS—that aren't always positive. "It can be pretty depressing," he quoted me, in an article that amounted to a manifesto about why environmental groups were unreasonably pessimistic.

Yes, it *can* be distressing to follow these trends. But now, with seven years under my Worldwatch belt, I have found that our work can quite often be inspirational.

For example, last spring, I wrote an op-ed for the *New York Times* encouraging Whole Foods, the largest natural and organic food seller in the world, to stock more produce, meat, and other products raised nearby. Whole Foods was about to open its third supermarket in Manhattan, across the street from the famed Union Square Greenmarket, New York's oldest and most legendary famers' market. Why not invite local growers to hand out samples during high-traffic shopping times, I suggested. Buy up excess produce at the end of the farmers' market. Feature New York produce in the store's prepared foods. Offer "all-New-York" catering options.

While researching the op-ed, the Whole Foods spokespeople I contacted were reluctant to say how much produce they planned to buy locally for their new store, even after I mentioned other New York supermarkets that made measurable commitments to supporting local farmers.

The op-ed came out a few days before the store opened, apparently without much of a splash and without any irate calls from Whole Foods executives. But several days later, a *Times* story on the opening quoted the same spokesperson I had interviewed—the commitment-phobe—as saying that the store "plans to buy up to 20 percent of its produce from farmers in the tristate region, some of whom also sell their food at the Greenmarket" and that "the chefs who cook the prepared foods at Whole Foods will shop in the Greenmarket and feature two to four Greenmarket specials daily."

It was a pleasant surprise, although I harbored no illusions that my op-ed prompted the change of heart. Buying local draws customers into stores and a smart company like Whole Foods could obviously see the writing on the wall. But, several weeks later, a Whole Foods "team leader" invited me to speak about the local foods movement at a Locally Grown Summit organized for staff in New York, New Jersey, and Connecticut.

The summit coincided with a new regional campaign the chain is planning that will involve building closer ties with nearby farmers, fishers, and food makers; educating staff on the benefits of buying local and educating customers on the benefits of eating local. (Among those ideas that came up during a brainstorm session—put staff in shirts saying "Ask me what's local," and develop interactive displays comparing the oil used to ship a Golden Delicious apple from New Zealand and a similar apple from the Northeast.)

It's too early to know what sort of success this program will enjoy, or what impact it will have on Whole Food's buying practices. But I recently got an e-mail from the president of a large Long Island food distributor that specializes in local produce: "Whole Foods contacted me after your article in the *Times* . . . They have requested I put a program together for them to procure more Long Island–grown produce. I have informed the Long Island Farm Bureau of the apparent success your article has had."

There have been other sources of inspiration. A marketing head of the largest food-service provider on Long Island contacted me to say they were rolling out a line of "Long Island Grown" selections for the chefs, cafeterias, and delis they supply, and that their shift was partly prompted by an employee who had read my book, *Eat Here*, which includes a chapter on the history and future of farming in my own area, the eastern end of Long Island. Last year, when I did a radio interview, one of the hosts mentioned that *Eat Here* had inspired people in the Anderson Valley to start a local food policy council and help steer local food politics. And, in the most immediate sign that my work hasn't been in vain, my wife and I have watched a farmers' market we launched in our hometown of Sag Harbor flourish as droves of locals come to enjoy fruit, vegetables, clams and oysters, mushrooms, raw-milk cheeses, jams, and honey raised by local artisans.

So, the work is not "depressing" and it isn't useless. In fact, although we at Worldwatch may not always know exactly how our work is being used, we do get glimpses and they give reason and hope to our work.

> Monsanto and DuPont control 90 percent of the commercially produced
> seeds in our country—they also brought us Agent Orange and stain-resistant
> carpet.

for Organic Lawn Care: Practices for the Design and Maintenance of Ecological Landscapes, which can be used as a resource by homeowners and professionals alike. From their perspective the best defense against unwanted weeds and insects is a healthy lawn. Pesticides can kill off beneficial insects and microorganisms that keep our lawns healthy, while healthy grass has better defenses against harmful weeds, insects, and microorganisms. Become familiar with the strengths and weaknesses of your soil and invest in building the healthiest environment for your lawn. Grass grows best in loamy soils with a mixture of clay, silt, sand, and plenty of organic matter on which to feed.

Here are NOFA's tips for a healthy, chemical-free lawn:

- Prepare a healthy soil. Many gardeners have their soil tested first by extension offices, to determine what its needs, if any, might be. A healthy soil and healthy lawn needs microorganisms and earthworms that decompose thatch and cuttings into nutrients for grass. Pesticides kill these helpful organisms, sterilizing your soil.
- If you're planting new grass, choose a variety that best suits your climate, sunlight, and rainfall or watering limitations.
- Don't assume that all weeds are the same. They could be rival grasses (bluegrass, crabgrass, Bermuda grass, quackgrass, chickweed), sedges (grasslike plants, including yellow nutsedge), or broadleaf plants (which have flat leaves, not needles or blades like grasses). Ground ivy, yellow woodsorrel, and white clover are some broadleaf perennials. Learn to distinguish weeds, and identify what you've got and how to fight it.
- Pull weeds when ground is moist, and then replant grass.
- Mow high and often. NOFA recommends a height of at least three inches. With more surface area, longer grass can absorb

more sunlight, which in turn allows a deeper root system to grow. Plus, weeds will have a harder time germinating with grass blocking the light.

- Mow with sharp blades to keep from shredding the grass. When you consider that an estimated 580 million gallons of gas are used each year to fuel lawn mowers, you may want to consider alternatives such as an old-fashioned push mower.

- According to the EPA, the average lawn consumes about 10,000 gallons of water annually beyond what it gets from rainfall. Nearly a third of all municipal water goes into irrigating lawns, according to the EPA. Water in the morning or evening to reduce evaporation loss and opt for longer, less frequent waterings so the water can really soak in.

- Break up the thatch with a rake or a machine. Thatch is dead plant material between the grass and the soil. Too much will create a barrier and prevent water from penetrating the soil. Healthy soil is full of earthworms and microorganisms that will help thatch decompose.

- Make sure there's proper drainage, and aerate during spring or fall. Aerating removes small cores from your lawn, allowing air and water to penetrate more deeply and benefit your lawn's root system.

Gardening

There is another way to live and think: It's called agrarianism. It is not so much a philosophy as a practice, an attitude, a loyalty, and a passion—all based in close connection with the land. It results in a sound local economy in which producers and consumers are neighbors and in which nature herself becomes the standard for work and production.

— WENDELL BERRY

Phillip Morris receives 10 cents of every dollar spent in grocery stores in this country, yet farmers receive only 9 cents of every food dollar spent.

Gardening, whether at home or in school, is one of the most important educational experiences we can share with our children. We believe that at different ages, children explore and interact with gardens differently. For instance, preschoolers may want to plant seeds, dig for worms, and even pluck strawberries or cherry tomatoes, but don't expect that they will make a strong connection between gardening and preparing food. Offer them the whole experience of food, flowers, and even some small animals, like rabbits and turtles. It's important that they feel comfortable on a farm or in a garden because it will set a tone for how they view gardening in the future. All they need is permission to explore the environment. What they learn about food in that setting will grow naturally out of their experience there.

As children get a bit older, say 5 or 6 years old, they may be able to use the garden as part of their "play." From storytelling to drawing to games like hide-and-seek, the garden can become a place of fantasy that unbridles the imagination. To allow this age group the most rewarding experiences, remember that food is grown in dirt and "dirty" is truly beautiful in this setting. Even eating some organic dirt on occasion is okay. Many of the elementary schools in Berkeley have school gardens, through grants from the California Nutrition Network and it's in these gardens where children really begin to be able plant and grow food. Garden lessons at this age can be about reading, writing, drawing, math, and science, as well as food, of course. Allow elementary school children to help pick out seeds to grow, help in the planting, and have watering and weeding be part of their "chores." Careful on the weeding—it's often difficult to tell the difference between the baby plant and the baby weed.

Martin Luther King Junior Middle School is home to The Edible Schoolyard in Berkeley, California. The grade levels at King are six, seven, and eight—and the students' abilities differ exponentially in the garden. Sixth graders are just beginning to be able to accomplish tasks

The Magic Garden Club

Summer is the best time for kids to get involved in gardening clubs or projects because there's so much to do—so much hands-on knowledge to acquire. At the Magic Garden Club in Falmouth, Massachusetts, kids ages 3½ to 6 have been getting their hands dirty for the last three years, and they love it!

In 2004 a mother of two and avid gardener, Sarah Pring, conceived a plan to offer "gardening adventure classes" at a nearby local farm. She chose forty varieties of organic seeds, including little finger carrots, Tom Thumb lettuce, yellow pear-shaped cherry tomatoes, scarlet runner beans, rainbow Swiss chard, and Black Beauty eggplant. Beginning in early June, children planted seeds and seedlings all over Peachtree Circle Farm, creating a sunflower snake, runner bean tepees, and a round pizza garden complete with basil plants. Each class made a couple of scarecrows and gave them names—Tyler Daisy was a particularly memorable straw-stuffed fellow. Flowers grew in an old bed frame, discarded boots, and virtually anything that would hold soil. On rainy days there were craft projects in the potting shed. As their plants matured, the children were allowed to pick herbs, vegetables, and flowers to take home and explore in their own kitchens with their families. A portion of the harvest was also shared with the Falmouth Service Center as part of the national "Plant a Row for the Hungry" initiative, and every class day, including when it rained, the children weeded, composted, and read garden-related stories designed to teach them about the farm's ecosystem. Throughout the season they kept journals, complete with photos, that became wonderful keepsakes of their summer in the garden. The end of the season was celebrated with a little harvest pizza party in late August.

In 2005 the Magic Garden Club partnered with the Cape Cod Children's Museum and moved to Coonamessett Farm, a larger, working farm with well-established community roots (and an ice-cream stand!). There, children were also exposed to a wide variety of animals, including alpacas and miniature Mediterranean donkeys. The program was so well-received by both children and parents that classes filled up with repeat business immediately. The per-child cost for 12 classes is roughly $200 and it's worth every penny. For more information about starting your own Magic Garden Club contact Sarah Pring at magicgardenclub @mac.com.

in the garden with a modicum of supervision. They can use tools, plant, harvest, and help to build structures in the garden—at Edible they can even harvest the freshly laid eggs. By the time students are at the end of middle school, they interact with the garden in a multidisciplinary fashion, from math to science to the business of selling the garden's harvest. They are at the age when they can be fully engaged in all aspects of gardening.

By high school, students can actively pursue all gardening and even many farming disciplines on their own. These young adults may be working in urban gardens growing food for themselves and their community, planning CSAs (Community-Supported Agriculture, see p. 192), or experimenting with hybrid or open-pollinated varieties of vegetables and fruits. One of the organizations that has become a model for gardening and farming with older children is the Food Project, based in Massachusetts. Begun in 1991, the Food Project has built a national reputation for engaging young people from diverse backgrounds in building a sustainable food system. Each year the organization works with more than a hundred teens and thousands of volunteers in growing more than 250,000 pounds of food without chemical pesticides. This food is then distributed to local shelters and through a CSA, farmers' markets, harvest bags, their own value-added products, and even catering. Seek out groups like this in your area to help your children find their passion for gardening.

Not all children will have the opportunity to participate in school or community gardens, but there are other creative ways to introduce kids to growing food—one of these is container gardening. The containers can be anything from window boxes to large metal or ceramic barrels, or even just plain plastic buckets. It doesn't matter which container you choose; the important thing is that you creatively engage children with growing food in nontraditional ways. You might have room on a windowsill, or perhaps you have a hallway with floor-to-ceiling south-facing windows. Your kitchen may have some light and space, or an entryway

Hog farms produce 1.3 billion tons of manure each year that is held in lagoons, often overflowing and contaminating rivers and polluting waters.

might turn out to be the perfect place. City dwellers may have room on a fire escape, or space in a room to add a grow light. Community and rooftop gardens are wonderful alternatives for urban children. One of the best resources for information on urban rooftop gardens is www.earth-pledge.com. The important thing to remember is that no matter where you are, you and your child can share the experience of growing food. Children can enjoy growing herbs and plants in almost any environment; as long as there is enough light and warmth anything is possible. For more information about container gardening look for *Container Gardening* by Patti Barrett (Storey Publishing, LLC, 1996).

No matter the type of garden you choose, you need to make sure that it is the safest possible environment for children. We strongly believe in organic gardening, using green growing techniques and organic inputs. This means that we recommend that you don't use synthetic chemicals, fertilizers, pesticides, or herbicides in your gardens, because there is some evidence that they are linked to cancer and should never be used where children are gardening.

Composting

At home or at school, two wonderful things you can share with children is composting and worm farming. Composting is the process of taking food and garden waste and allowing it to decompose to the point where it actually becomes nutrient-rich material (aka dirt) that will augment our garden's soil while relieving the pressure on our landfills and waste management systems. Compost can be spread onto gardens or mixed in with soils that need enhancing. Nutrients found in compost eventually become part of the plant. Research by Rodale and others shows that vegetables grown in nutrient-rich soils, often as part of an organic system, have significantly more nutrients than the same vegetables grown in a conventional system with synthetic nitrogen-based fertilizers.

There is a wide variety of composting systems available to gardeners, the most basic of which involves a pile of food waste layered with shredded paper or hay. With this method there is a bit of manual labor, but the resulting compost is as rich and dense as compost derived by any other method. In other words, you don't need to spend money on a spinning drum or plastic bin to make composting work for you. The Earth Machine, one of our favorites because of its ease and simplicity, can be found at www.composters.com.

Another delightfully educational experience for children that benefits the garden is worm farming. In our experience most kids love worms and "farming" them at home or at school is a great way to learn about the cycle of food waste. It's a simple way of processing food waste into soil or a nutritional soil amendment. There are a number of packaged starter kits that you can use, but you might also choose to make your own out of wood or even plastic containers. After you make or buy a container, all you have to do is purchase some worms (red worms are the preferred variety) and start feeding them food scraps mixed with recycled paper scraps (black and white only—no color prints). Keep them warm and fed and they'll create soil from your food waste. For urbanites and those without the yard space for a compost system, worm farming might prove the perfect food waste tool. For more information check out www.wormdigest.org.

Conservation

In our country we are losing farmland at the alarming rate of two acres a minute. We must reverse this trend or delicious local, seasonal food will become a thing of the past. A number of groups are helping out by supporting local farms, farmers' markets, and farmers, and we encourage you to support these nonprofit organizations by lending a hand or making tax-deductible donations.

America is losing farmland at the rate of 2 acres per minute.

More than 30 percent of the food produced for human consumption is thrown out as waste.

Quail Hill Farm in Amagansett, New York, is a working farm and CSA run by Scott Chaskey. It is being preserved by the Nature Conservancy, which was founded more than fifty years ago and whose mission it is "to preserve the plants and natural communities that represent the diversity of life on Earth by protecting the lands and waters they need to survive." In fact, the Nature Conservancy has protected more than 100 million acres of land and 5,000 miles of river in all fifty states and twenty-seven other countries.

American Farmland Trust (AFT) is another advocacy group working to save farms and farmers. Founded in 1980, the Trust has helped to win permanent protection for more than a million acres of American farmland that might otherwise have become roads, houses, or malls. AFT works to protect land through publicly funded conservation easement programs, plans for growth of acreage in agriculture lands through community planning, and works toward keeping the land healthy by encouraging stewardship and conservation.

We hope that you feel, as we do, that supporting these types of initiatives is something you can do. For more information see our resource guide on page 223.

"When you wake up in the morning, Pooh," said Piglet at last, "what's the first thing you say to yourself?"
"What's for breakfast?" said Pooh. "What do you say, Piglet?"
"I say, I wonder what's going to happen exciting today?" said Piglet.
Pooh nodded thoughtfully.
"It's the same thing," he said.

—A.A. MILNE

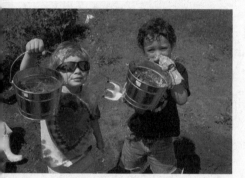

CHAPTER 4

Breakfast and Snacks

We know you've heard it before, but breakfast really is the most important meal of the day. Studies like the one conducted by Harvard University and Massachusetts General Hospital show that children perform better on standardized tests, exhibit less hyperactivity, and generally behave better than kids who skip breakfast.[1] And while eating breakfast at all is bet-

[1]"Relationship Between Hunger and Psychosocial Functioning in Low-Income American Children," Murphy, J. Michael EdD; Wehler, Cheryl A. MS; Pagano, Maria E. EdM; Little, Michelle BA; Kleinman, Ronald E. MD; Jellinek, Michael S. MD, *Journal of the American Academy of Child and Adolescent Psychiatry*, February, 1998.

Weeding at the Magic Garden Club in Falmouth, Massachusetts *Sarah Pring*

ter than no breakfast, the kinds of foods your kids eat in the morning will affect them for the rest of the day. A breakfast high in sugar, one Oxford University study suggests, may actually make them feel like eating lunches with more calories than they need.[2] Even if you have a limited amount of time in the morning it's still possible to put something healthful together.

Snacks are also an important part of every child's day and with a little planning you can make some tasty, nutritionally sound snacks for your kids with little effort. The Apple Date Bars featured in this chapter are delicious and easy to make. Fruit Smoothies (page 148) are always a big hit with kids, and there's a list of quick snacks (see page 152) for those days when you're short on time so you don't fall into the sugared snack trap. Whole foods like fruits and nuts will give your children the energy boost they need without the empty calories sugar provides.

A Note on Using the Recipes Included in This Book

Calorie Needs and Serving Sizes

The USDA bases its Nutrition Facts labeling on a 2000-calorie diet. For the sake of consistency we have done the same in this book. However, for most children, the serving size will differ from what the USDA uses as its median guideline. To make things easier for you when trying to determine serving sizes for your children we suggest that you use the following conversion factors as a general guideline:

CHILD'S AGE	MULTIPLY SERVING SIZE, CALORIES, AND DAILY VALUES BY:
6 months to 1 year	0.42
2 to 6 years	0.8
Any child between 7 and 12 years *as well as* teen girls	1.1
Teen boys	1.4

[2] "Low Glycemic Index Breakfasts and Reduced Food Intake in Preadolescent Children," Warren, Janet M. PhD; Henry, C. Jeya K. PhD; Simonite, Vanessa, PhD, *Pediatrics*, November 2003.

SAMPLE CONVERSIONS:

Breakfast Polenta Casserole

USDA NATIONAL AVERAGE

NUTRITION FACTS

Serving Size: 1 serving (28g/1oz.) ■ Servings Per Recipe: 8 ■ Amount Per Serving ■ Calories: 334 ■ Calories from fat: 165 (49% of tot cal) ■ % Daily Value* ■ Total Fat 18g 28% ■ Saturated Fat 9g 44% ■ Cholesterol 189mg 63% ■ Sodium 486mg 20% ■ Total Carbo 23g 8% ■ Dietary Fiber 2g 8% ■ Sugars 21g ■ Protein 17g ■ Vitamin A 49% ■ Vitamin C 16% ■ Calcium 30% ■ Iron 19% ■ 2000 calorie diet

CHILDREN 6 MONTHS TO 1 YEAR

NUTRITION FACTS

Serving Size: 1 serving (12g/.4oz.) ■ Servings Per Recipe: 19 ■ Amount Per Serving ■ Calories: 134 ■ Calories from fat: 66 (49% of tot cal) ■ % Daily Value* ■ Total Fat 7g 28% ■ Saturated Fat 4g 44% ■ Cholesterol 76mg 63% ■ Sodium 194mg 20% ■ Total Carbo 9g 8% ■ Dietary Fiber 1g 8% ■ Sugars 8g ■ Protein 7g ■ Vitamin A 49% ■ Vitamin C 16% ■ Calcium 30% ■ Iron 19% ■ 850 calorie diet

CHILDREN 2 TO 6 YEARS

NUTRITION FACTS

Serving Size: 1 serving (22g/.8oz.) ■ Servings Per Recipe: 10 ■ Amount Per Serving ■ Calories: 267 ■ Calories from fat: 132 (49% of tot cal) ■ % Daily Value* ■ Total Fat 14g 28% ■ Saturated Fat 7g 44% ■ Cholesterol 151mg 63% ■ Sodium 389mg 20% ■ Total Carbo 18g 8% ■ Dietary Fiber 2g 8% ■ Sugars 17g ■ Protein 14g ■ Vitamin A 49% ■ Vitamin C 16% ■ Calcium 30% ■ Iron 19% ■ 1600 calorie diet

CHILDREN 7 TO 12 YEARS AND TEEN GIRLS

NUTRITION FACTS

Serving Size: 1 serving (31g/1.1oz.) ■ Servings Per Recipe: 7 ■ Amount Per Serving ■ Calories: 367 ■ Calories from fat: 182 (49% of tot cal) ■ % Daily Value* ■ Total Fat 20g 28% ■ Saturated Fat 10g 44% ■ Cholesterol 208mg 63% ■ Sodium 535mg 20% ■ Total Carbo 25g 8% ■ Dietary Fiber 2g 8% ■ Sugars 23g ■ Protein 19g ■ Vitamin A 49% ■ Vitamin C 16% ■ Calcium 30% ■ Iron 19% ■ 2200 calorie diet

TEEN BOYS

NUTRITION FACTS

Serving Size: 1 serving (39g/1.4oz.) ■ Servings Per Recipe: 6 ■ Amount Per Serving ■ Calories: 468 ■ Calories from fat: 231 (49% of tot cal) ■ % Daily Value* ■ Total Fat 25g 28% ■ Saturated Fat 13g 44% ■ Cholesterol 265mg 63% ■ Sodium 680mg 20% ■ Total Carbo 32g 8% ■ Dietary Fiber 3g 8% ■ Sugars 29g ■ Protein 24g ■ Vitamin A 49% ■ Vitamin C 16% ■ Calcium 30% ■ Iron 19% ■ 2800 calorie diet

KEY TO RECIPES

 lunch box easy

 keep it hot in a wide-mouth vacuum bottle

CPF—Chez Panisse Foundation

R—Ross School

FB—FullBloom Baking Company

FC—FoodChange

Banana Bread R

■

8 SERVINGS

Did you know that banana trees produce one large beautiful flower and only one bunch of (several dozen) bananas a year? Amazing when you consider that 85 million tons of bananas are consumed around the world annually. Bananas are a labor-intensive industry, much of which is done by hand: From hauling banana "trains" of 25- to 100-pound bunches to sorting for size and quality, almost all banana production is done by hand.

Children of all ages seem to love the flavor and texture of bananas, and banana bread is a great way to utilize your overripe bananas. Two tips: Conventionally grown bananas are loaded with pesticides, so buy organic whenever possible. Also, bananas may be peeled and frozen in plastic bags so you can save extras until you have enough to make a full recipe.

butter, to grease the pan
¾ cup cake flour
¼ cup all-purpose flour
¼ teaspoon baking powder
¼ teaspoon baking soda
¼ teaspoon kosher salt
¼ teaspoon ground cinnamon
⅛ teaspoon ground cloves
½ cup sugar
¼ cup nonfat yogurt
¼ cup sour cream
2 tablespoons (¼ stick) unsalted butter
¼ teaspoon vanilla extract
1 large egg
2 very ripe medium bananas, mashed

1. Preheat oven to 350°F and grease an 8 × 4-inch loaf pan with butter.
2. Sift together the flours, baking powder, baking soda, salt, cinnamon, and cloves and set aside.
3. Cream the sugar, yogurt, sour cream, butter, and vanilla together in a mixer using the paddle attachment, scraping down the sides of the bowl. Add the egg and mix again.
4. When the egg is fully incorporated, add small amounts of the sifted dry ingredients, mixing between additions.
5. Finish by adding the mashed bananas. Do not overmix or the bread will be dense and heavy; mix only until all ingredients are incorporated.
6. Pour batter into the prepared pan and bake for 30 to 40 minutes. Use a toothpick to test for doneness. Allow to cool before slicing.

NUTRITION FACTS

Serving Size: 1-inch slice ■ Servings Per Recipe: 8 ■ Amount Per Serving ■ Calories: 177 ■ Calories from fat: 48 (25% of tot cal) ■ % Daily Value* ■ Total Fat 5g 8% ■ Saturated Fat 3g 15% ■ Cholesterol 42mg 14% ■ Sodium 144mg 6% ■ Total Carbo 29g 10% ■ Dietary Fiber 1g 3% ■ Sugars 15g ■ Protein 3g ■ Vitamin A 22% ■ Vitamin C 3% ■ Calcium 5% ■ Iron 13%

*Percent Daily Values are based on a 2000 calorie diet. Your daily values may be higher or lower depending upon your caloric intake.

Low-Fat Oat-Fruit Scone FB

16 SERVINGS

FullBloom Baking Company is owned by an amazing woman, Karen Trilevsky, who worked for months with the help of her team to develop recipes for the pilot universal breakfast program in the Berkeley Unified School District. This is one of her recipes. Fresh and dried fruits work equally well in these scones, as do nuts. Let your kids suggest their favorite fruit and/or nut combinations and try these more than once.

1 egg

1 cup buttermilk

3 tablespoons canola oil

2 teaspoons grated orange zest

1/2 cup rolled oats

1 1/2 cups whole-wheat flour

1 1/2 cups all-purpose flour

1/3 cup raw sugar

1 tablespoon baking powder

1 teaspoon salt

2 1/2 cups fruit and/or nuts (berries, cherries, peaches, raisins, etc.)

1. Preheat the oven to 350°F. Grease a cookie sheet with spray oil and set aside.
2. Beat the egg in a small bowl and mix well with the buttermilk.
3. Add the canola oil and orange zest and mix to combine.
4. In a large bowl, mix together the oats, flours, sugar, baking powder, and salt.
5. Stir the buttermilk mixture into the dry ingredients and mix just until the dough comes together. Do not overmix.
6. Fold in the fruit and/or nuts.
7. Scoop heaping tablespoons of the dough onto the prepared cookie sheet and bake 10 minutes or until slightly golden on top.

NUTRITION FACTS

Serving Size: 1 scone ■ Servings Per Recipe: 16 ■ Amount Per Serving ■ Calories: 153 ■ Calories from fat: 32 (20% of tot cal) ■ % Daily Value* ■ Total Fat 4g 5% ■ Saturated Fat 0g 2% ■ Cholesterol 16mg 5% ■ Sodium 237mg 10% ■ Total Carbo 27g 10% ■ Dietary Fiber 3g 10% ■ Sugars 7g ■ Protein 4g ■ Vitamin A 17% ■ Vitamin C 5% ■ Calcium 10% ■ Iron 13%

*Percent Daily Values are based on a 2000 calorie diet. Your daily values may be higher or lower depending upon your caloric intake.

Three Cheese–Vegetable Strata R

8 SERVINGS

Ever wonder what to do with all your stale, leftover bread or bread ends? This recipe provides a solution that can be made the night before for an easy early morning start. Feel free to experiment with other vegetables and/or leftover meats and sausage for a more protein-rich alternative.

> "IT IS DELICIOUS!!!!! The recipe was easy to follow
> and I could eat the whole pan!!"
>
> —MICHELLE WIESNER, AURORA, CO, MOTHER OF FOUR

2½ tablespoons unsalted butter, plus extra for the pan
3 cups (1 lb.) button mushrooms, cleaned and sliced
1 cup Spanish onion (1 medium), diced small
3 cups sliced asparagus (1 bunch, 1-inch slices)
6 slices sourdough bread, crust removed, diced large
¼ cup shredded Cheddar cheese
¼ cup crumbled goat cheese
¼ cup grated Parmesan cheese
3 large eggs
1¼ cups milk
½ teaspoon salt
Freshly ground black pepper

1. *The night before:* Butter a 9 × 9-inch baking dish.
2. In a heavy skillet, melt the butter and sauté the mushrooms and onion for 2 minutes. When tender, add the asparagus and sauté for 1 minute.

3. Layer the bread, the mushroom mixture, and the cheeses into the prepared baking dish.

4. Combine the eggs, milk, and salt in a small bowl and whisk until well blended. Season with salt and pepper to taste. Pour the egg mixture over the mushroom mixture, cover, and refrigerate overnight.

5. *The next morning:* Preheat oven to 350°F.

6. Bake for about 40 minutes or until the top begins to brown and the eggs are firm.

7. Remove from the oven and let stand for a few minutes before cutting.

NUTRITION FACTS

Serving Size: One 3 × 3-inch square ■ Servings Per Recipe: 8 ■ Amount Per Serving ■ Calories: 269 ■ Calories from fat: 110 (40% of tot cal) ■ % Daily Value* ■ Total Fat 11g 17% ■ Saturated Fat 7g 33% ■ Cholesterol 117mg 39% ■ Sodium 569mg 24% ■ Total Carbo 25g 9% ■ Dietary Fiber 3g 12% ■ Sugars 3g ■ Protein 15g ■ Vitamin A 82% ■ Vitamin C 21% ■ Calcium 27% ■ Iron 24%

*Percent Daily Values are based on a 2000 calorie diet. Your daily values may be higher or lower depending upon your caloric intake.

Yogurt-Honey Health Muffins R

■

24 MINI-MUFFINS

The addition of yogurt not only makes these muffins moist and nutritionally sound, but helps them stay fresh in an airtight container for up to three days and still taste wonderful. If cake flour is not readily available, all-purpose flour can be substituted. The muffins will be slightly denser, but will taste just as good.

1½ cups cake flour

1 teaspoon baking powder

1 teaspoon baking soda

¾ teaspoon kosher salt

4½ teaspoons sugar

2 tablespoons rolled oats

1 tablespoon diced dried cranberries

1 tablespoon diced dried apricots

1 tablespoon unsalted sunflower seeds

1 teaspoon grated orange zest

1 tablespoon toasted bran

½ cup nonfat yogurt

¼ cup honey

1 teaspoon vanilla extract

8 tablespoons (1 stick) unsalted butter, melted

2 large eggs

1. Preheat the oven to 350°F and grease a mini-muffin pan.
2. In a large mixing bowl, sift together the flour, baking powder, baking soda, salt, and sugar. Add the oats, dried fruits, sunflower seeds, orange zest, and bran and mix to combine.
3. In another bowl, combine the yogurt, honey, vanilla, butter, and eggs and stir until the ingredients are well blended. Pour the yogurt mixture into the dry ingredients and stir to mix, just until all ingredients are incorporated. Take care not to overmix.
4. Fill muffin cups two-thirds of the way with batter. Bake for approximately 20 minutes or until golden.

NUTRITION FACTS
Serving Size: 1 mini-muffin ■ Servings Per Recipe: 24 ■ Amount Per Serving ■ Calories: 95 ■ Calories from fat: 42 (44% of tot cal) ■ % Daily Value* ■ Total Fat 5g 7% ■ Saturated Fat 3g 13% ■ Cholesterol 31mg 10% ■ Sodium 191mg 8% ■ Total Carbo 12g 4% ■ Dietary Fiber 0g 1% ■ Sugars 5g ■ Protein 2g ■ Vitamin A 19% ■ Vitamin C 0% ■ Calcium 3% ■ Iron 8%

*Percent Daily Values are based on a 2000 calorie diet. Your daily values may be higher or lower depending upon your caloric intake.

12-Grain Muffins FB

24 MINI-MUFFINS

These muffins were developed by FullBloom for the pilot Universal Breakfast program in the Berkeley Unified School District, that began in the spring of 2004. They are healthy, delicious, and nutritious, and are a great component of breakfast. Serve with your child's favorite flavored yogurt and breakfast will surely be a hit. Like the other muffins we feature, these freeze well. In fact, freezing is preferable to refrigeration if you want to save them for more than a couple of days because it locks moisture in, while refrigeration dries foods out.

Ben Holmes yelled out, "Look, Mom, Kaia LOVES that muffin!" as his 10-month-old sister tried to shove the entire muffin in her mouth at once.

½ cup 12-grain cereal (or 10-grain cereal if 12-grain isn't available)

1 cup boiling water

½ cup chopped dates

1 teaspoon salt

¼ cup honey

2 tablespoons maple syrup

1 large egg

¼ cup canola oil

½ cup buttermilk

1 cup whole-wheat flour

2 teaspoons baking powder

1 teaspoon baking soda

1 teaspoon ground cinnamon

1 cup chopped raw mixed seeds and nuts such as pumpkin, sesame, flax, sunflower, walnut, cashews

1. *The night before:* Combine the cereal, boiling water, dates, and salt in a small bowl. Soak, covered for 8 hours.
2. *The next day:* Preheat oven to 350°F and grease a mini-muffin pan.
3. In a small bowl, combine the honey, maple syrup, egg, oil, and buttermilk, and set aside.
4. In a medium bowl combine the flour, baking powder, baking soda, and cinnamon and mix well.
5. Mix the cereal mixture into wet ingredients and then add to the dry ingredients, stirring only until combined.
6. Scoop into muffin cups. Sprinkle the tops with a mixture of colorful seeds and nuts.
7. Bake in a 350°F oven approximately 20 minutes, or until a toothpick comes out clean.

NUTRITION FACTS

Serving Size: 1 mini-muffin ▪ Servings Per Recipe: 24 ▪ Amount Per Serving ▪ Calories: 88 ▪ Calories from fat: 30 (34% of tot cal) ▪ % Daily Val ▪ Total Fat 3g 5% ▪ Saturated Fat 1g 2% ▪ Cholesterol 10mg 3% ▪ Sodium 191mg 8% ▪ Total Carbo 15g 5% ▪ Dietary Fiber 1g 5% ▪ Sugars 7g ▪ Protein 2g ▪ Vitamin A 12% ▪ Vitamin C 3% ▪ Calcium 5% ▪ Iron 9%

*Percent Daily Values are based on a 2000 calorie diet. Your daily values may be higher or lower depending upon your caloric intake.

Breakfast Burritos with Tofu R

8 SERVINGS

Breakfast burritos are a warm and filling start to the day. This is a meal that can be packed to go if time is limited, or even eaten later in the day for lunch. If tofu isn't your thing, scramble in a couple of eggs or fry up a few pieces of turkey bacon for added protein. In too much of a hurry to wait for the potatoes to cook? Leave them out or chop up a leftover baked potato and you'll only have to sauté it until heated through.

¾ cup Spanish onion (1 medium), diced small

1 clove garlic, minced

1 tablespoon canola oil

1½ cups potatoes, diced medium

1 teaspoon kosher salt

½ teaspoon freshly ground black pepper

½ pound firm tofu, diced medium

8 6-inch flour tortillas

1¼ cups fat-free refried beans

1½ cups (6 ounces) shredded Monterey Jack cheese

½ cup Tomato Salsa (page 129)

1. Over medium heat, sauté the onion and garlic in oil in a large skillet until the onions are translucent, about 2 minutes. Add the potatoes, salt, and pepper. Cook until potatoes are tender and browned. Add the tofu and heat gently.
2. Fill the center of each tortilla with refried beans, the potato/tofu mixture, and the cheese.
3. Roll up the tortillas and top each one with a spoonful of salsa. If the burrito is going to be eaten on the run put the salsa inside the tortilla. For lunch, send the salsa on the side so the tortilla doesn't get soggy.

NUTRITION FACTS

Serving Size: 1 burrito ■ Servings Per Recipe: 8 ■ Amount Per Serving ■ Calories: 265 ■ Calories from fat: 56 (21% of tot cal) ■ % Daily Value* ■ Total Fat 6g 10% ■ Saturated Fat 0g 2% ■ Cholesterol 3mg 1% ■ Sodium 884mg 37% ■ Total Carbo 43g 14% ■ Dietary Fiber 3g 14% ■ Sugars 2g ■ Protein 10g ■ Vitamin A 17% ■ Vitamin C 35% ■ Calcium 15% ■ Iron 27%

*Percent Daily Values are based on a 2000 calorie diet. Your daily values may be higher or lower depending upon your caloric intake.

The Institute of Medicine and the National Association for Sports and Physical Education recommend that children accumulate a minimum of 60 minutes of physical activity a day.

Quick Tips for Dealing with a Picky Eater

1. Make sure you set a good example. If you turn your nose up at certain foods, you can't expect your child to try them, either.

2. Talk about what good nutrition is and make sure that you explain to your child that she needs a variety of foods in her diet. Show her the Healthy Meal Wheel and explain the importance of each type of food.

3. Let your child help with food shopping and preparation. Kids like to eat what they make, but you also might learn something new about why he likes or doesn't like certain foods.

4. Since it takes time for kids to warm up to new foods, require at least a one-bite minimum (not a tip-of-the-tongue taste, a real, in-the-mouth bite) to make sure she's at least trying something new. She may be pleasantly surprised.

5. Offer choices, but keep them limited. Don't just ask what your child wants for lunch, but give him two or three concrete options—pasta salad, a tuna sandwich, or a square of leftover lasagna?

6. Reward children with a sticker on a chart if they try new foods. Don't get upset if they refuse to try something.

7. Try different preparations of the same food. Sometimes just a change in the way things look makes all the difference to a kid.

8. Serve age- and size-appropriate portions. The volume of things on a plate may be enough to turn a kid off.

9. Limit snacks and drinks for several hours before a meal. Some children will fill up on snacks before dinner especially, and simply are not hungry when it's time to sit down and eat. They may seem like picky eaters, but they're really just full.

10. Don't allow yourself to fall into a power struggle over food with your child. It will never be helpful and may even be detrimental.

Tomato Salsa R

8 SERVINGS

Salsa is a great way to add flavor and spice to all sorts of meals. Think beyond Mexican and use salsas to add robust flavor to grilled and roasted chicken, pork, and beef. Even scrambled eggs benefit from a healthy dose of salsa!

1 pound Roma tomatoes, diced medium

2 teaspoons chopped fresh cilantro

2½ teaspoons seeded and chopped jalapeño pepper

1 cup red onion (1 medium), diced small

3 tablespoons lime juice

2 teaspoons kosher salt

½ teaspoon freshly ground black pepper

Mix all ingredients together and marinate for 20 to 30 minutes. Refrigerate leftovers for up to 1 week.

NUTRITION FACTS

Serving Size: 6 tablespoons ■ Servings Per Recipe: 8 ■ Amount Per Serving ■ Calories: 22 ■ Calories from fat: 2 (1% of tot cal) ■ % Daily Value* ■ Total Fat 0g 0% ■ Saturated Fat 0g 0% ■ Cholesterol 0mg 0% ■ Sodium 595mg 25% ■ Total Carbo 5g 2% ■ Dietary Fiber 1g 4% ■ Sugars 1g ■ Protein 1g ■ Vitamin A 37% ■ Vitamin C 41% ■ Calcium 1% ■ Iron 4%

*Percent Daily Values are based on a 2000 calorie diet. Your daily values may be higher or lower depending upon your caloric intake.

 About half of U.S. schools require physical education for children grades 1 through 5; however, fewer than 10 percent of high schools require physical education for students in grades 10 to 12.

Frittata with Spinach, Mushrooms, and Cheese R

8 SERVINGS

A frittata is the best kind of omelet because there's no flipping involved. We make them in cast-iron pans and bring them to the table right in the pan where we cut them like a pie. Don't like spinach or mushrooms? Substitute your seasonal favorites.

12 large eggs, beaten
2 teaspoons kosher salt
1/2 teaspoon freshly ground black pepper
1 1/2 teaspoons vegetable oil
1 1/2 teaspoons unsalted butter
1 3/4 cups sliced crimini mushrooms
1/2 cup (4 ounces) shredded Cheddar cheese
1 cup blanched spinach, chopped

1. Preheat oven to 300°F. Season the beaten eggs with the salt and pepper.
2. Warm a large ovenproof skillet over medium heat. The pan should not get too hot. Add the oil and butter and sauté the mushrooms, remove and reserve. Pour in eggs to form the base of the frittata.
3. When the eggs begin to cook, place the cooked mushrooms and the spinach on the frittata, taking care to distribute evenly.
4. Transfer to the oven. The frittata will be done when the top begins to brown and the eggs are fluffy, 5 minutes or so.

NUTRITION FACTS

Serving Size: 1/8 of the frittata ■ Servings Per Recipe: 8 ■ Amount Per Serving ■ Calories: 140 ■ Calories from fat: 95 (68% of tot cal) ■ %Daily Value* ■ Total Fat 11g 16% ■ Saturated Fat 5g 26% ■ Cholesterol

204mg 68% ■ Sodium 753mg 31% ■ Total Carbo 1g 0% ■ Dietary Fiber 0g 2% ■ Sugars 1g ■ Protein 10g ■ Vitamin A 98% ■ Vitamin C 6% ■ Calcium 15% ■ Iron 11%

*Percent Daily Values are based on a 2000 calorie diet. Your daily values may be higher or lower depending upon your caloric intake.

■:

Breakfast Polenta Casserole R

■

8 SERVINGS

The flavors and textures of corn polenta are warmly comforting. Whether in this casserole, served as a hot breakfast cereal either sweet or savory, or as a side dish with an entrée, this grain can become part of any healthy meal. This recipe can be done on the same day if you have time, but if you know you're going to be pressed for time, preparing some of it the night before is helpful.

Olive oil

¼ cup red onion (1 small), diced small

1¼ cup unpeeled Yukon gold potatoes (1 large), diced small

Salt

Freshly ground black pepper

6 ounces raw pork sausage, casings removed

3 cups water

1 cup coarse cornmeal or polenta

5 large eggs

butter or oil for sauteeing

½ cup grated Parmesan cheese

⅔ cup shredded sharp Cheddar cheese

1. *The night before:* Heat a small amount of olive oil in a medium skillet and sauté the onions over medium-low heat until golden

brown. While the onions are cooking, steam the potatoes in a small amount of water in a covered pot until they are tender. Drain.

2. Add the steamed potatoes to the onions, season with salt and pepper, and cook the potato-onion mixture until the potatoes are browned. Set aside in a covered bowl.

3. Cook the sausage, breaking it up as it cooks, until it is no longer pink. Drain and cool.

4. Refrigerate the onion-potato mixture and the sausage separately overnight.

5. *The next morning:* Preheat the oven to 350°F.

6. To prepare the polenta, bring 3 cups of water to a boil. Whisk in the cornmeal and cook the mixture over low heat, stirring occasionally, until thick and smooth (approximately 7 minutes).

7. Pour the polenta into an ungreased baking dish. It will begin to get firm as you scramble the eggs.

8. Beat the eggs in a small bowl and season with salt and pepper. Heat butter or oil in a skillet over medium heat. Pour in the eggs and scramble them until slightly firm but still wet. Remove from the heat. (The eggs will finish cooking in the oven.)

9. Spread the potato mixture, sausage, Parmesan, and Cheddar over the polenta. Pour the eggs on top of the entire dish. Bake until heated through and the cheese is melted and bubbly.

10. Cool slightly, then cut and serve.

NUTRITION FACTS

Serving Size: About 8 ounces ■ Servings Per Recipe: 8 ■ Amount Per Serving ■ Calories: 334 ■ Calories from fat: 178 (53% of tot cal) ■ %Daily Value* ■ Total Fat 20g 30% ■ Saturated Fat 9g 44% ■ Cholesterol 189mg 63% ■ Sodium 486mg 20% ■ Total Carbo 21g 7% ■ Dietary Fiber 2g 8% ■ Sugars 1g ■ Protein 17g ■ Vitamin A 49% ■ Vitamin C 16% ■ Calcium 30% ■ Iron 19%

*Percent Daily Values are based on a 2000 calorie diet. Your daily values may be higher or lower depending upon your caloric intake.

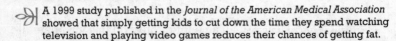 A 1999 study published in the *Journal of the American Medical Association* showed that simply getting kids to cut down the time they spend watching television and playing video games reduces their chances of getting fat.

Scrambled Eggs with Spinach, Chives, and Goat Cheese R

8 SERVINGS

Nothing is better than farm-fresh eggs. When Ann worked at the Ross School she was fortunate to have Iocona Farms as a purveyor of fresh chicken and eggs. The Ross School served hundreds of dozens of Iocona's eggs over the years, and this recipe was a school favorite. When shopping for eggs go for the brown ones to help support biodiversity in the food supply. This is important for one reason: All white eggs are laid by one variety of chicken, the White Leghorn, and most of our eggs are white. If there's a devastating disease that kills White Leghorn chickens we'd be facing a huge egg shortage similar to Ireland's great potato famine. Brown eggs aren't necessarily healthier for your body, but they're healthier for the longevity of the country's egg supply. If you have leftovers save and reheat them in the microwave. They're great wrapped in a tortilla.

6 cups fresh spinach, heavy stems removed

16 large eggs

1/2 teaspoon kosher salt

1/8 teaspoon freshly ground black pepper

2 tablespoons olive oil

1/4 pound (about 1/2 cup) goat cheese, crumbled

2 tablespoons chopped chives

1. Bring a large pot of salted water to a boil. Drop in the spinach and cook just until wilted. Drain in a colander and cool under cold running water. Squeeze out excess liquid and chop.
2. Beat the eggs well in a medium bowl and season with the salt and pepper.

3. Heat the oil in a skillet, preferably nonstick. Pour in the eggs and cook over medium heat until eggs begin to set.
4. Add the spinach, cheese, and chives and continue cooking until the eggs are set, but still soft. Serve hot.

NUTRITION FACTS

Serving Size: About 1 cup ■ Servings Per Recipe: 8 ■ Amount Per Serving ■ Calories: 269 ■ Calories from fat: 176% (65% of tot cal) ■ % Daily Value* ■ Total Fat 20g 30% ■ Saturated Fat 7g 35% ■ Cholesterol 504mg 168% ■ Sodium 411mg 17% ■ Total Carbo 3g 1% ■ Dietary Fiber 2g 6% ■ Sugars 2g ■ Protein 19g ■ Vitamin A 476% ■ Vitamin C 36% ■ Calcium 17% ■ Iron 35%

*Percent Daily Values are based on a 2000 calorie diet. Your daily values may be higher or lower depending upon your caloric intake.

Peanut Butter and Jelly Power Muffins R

20 MINI-MUFFINS

PB & J is a favorite for just about every kid. It's no wonder then that this would be such a popular muffin with children. A "healthy" muffin, it can be made ahead and stored in the freezer for up to two weeks. To defrost just remove from the freezer and bring to room temperature, then store in an airtight container for up to 3 days.

1 cup whole-wheat flour

1½ teaspoons baking powder

1 teaspoon baking soda

½ teaspoon kosher salt

½ cup maple sugar

1 teaspoon ground cinnamon

6 tablespoons rolled oats

3 tablespoons raisins

¼ cup chopped raw peanuts

½ cup soy milk

4 tablespoons canola oil

6 tablespoons maple syrup

1 teaspoon vanilla extract

½ cup peanut butter

1 tablespoon cider vinegar

2 medium bananas, mashed

4 tablespoons strawberry jam

1. Preheat the oven to 350°F and grease a mini-muffin pan.
2. Into a large mixing bowl, sift together the flour, baking powder, baking soda, salt, maple sugar, and cinnamon. Add the oats, raisins, and half of the peanuts.
3. In another bowl, combine the soy milk, oil, maple syrup, vanilla, peanut butter, vinegar, and bananas and mash until the ingredients are well blended, then pour into the dry ingredients, stirring to mix just until all ingredients are incorporated. Take care not to overmix.
4. Fill muffin cups two-thirds full with batter, then drop a little jam onto the top of each muffin. Sprinkle the tops with the remaining peanuts and bake for approximately 20 minutes, until a toothpick comes out clean.

NUTRITION FACTS

Serving Size: 1 mini-muffin ▪ Servings Per Recipe: 20 ▪ Amount Per Serving ▪ Calories: 96 ▪ Calories from fat: 46 (48% of tot cal) ▪ % Daily Value* ▪ Total Fat 5g 8% ▪ Saturated Fat 1g 4% ▪ Cholesterol 0mg 0% ▪ Sodium 91mg 4% ▪ Total Carbo 11g 4% ▪ Dietary Fiber 1g 3% ▪ Sugars 5g ▪ Protein 3g ▪ Vitamin A 0% ▪ Vitamin C 1% ▪ Calcium 3% ▪ Iron 6%

*Percent Daily Values are based on a 2000 calorie diet. Your daily values may be higher or lower depending upon your caloric intake.

 BBC News reported in 2005 that children aged 11 to 15 now spend 53 hours a week—7½ hours a day—watching TV and sitting in front of computers, an increase of 40 percent in a decade.

Granola R

▪

1 POUND

Homemade is always better than store-bought—and granola is easy to make. Double or triple this recipe, put it in plastic storage bags, and freeze it for up to 3 months. To thaw, just remove the granola from the freezer and bring it to room temperature. Store thawed granola in an airtight container. This recipe is not only great for breakfast, but in a smaller portion is a wonderful mid-afternoon snack or side dish in a lunch box.

2 teaspoons unsalted butter

1 tablespoon + 1½ teaspoons canola oil

1 tablespoon honey

2 tablespoons + 1½ teaspoons maple syrup

1¾ cup rolled oats

¾ cup toasted unsweetened coconut

½ teaspoon salt

¼ teaspoon ground cinnamon

¼ cup toasted whole unsalted almonds

¼ cup toasted unsalted pumpkin seeds

1 tablespoon toasted unsalted sunflower seeds

¼ cup raisins

1 tablespoon golden raisins

¼ cup dried cherries

1 tablespoon dried apricots, diced small

1. Preheat oven to 200°F.
2. In a small saucepan, heat the butter, oil, honey, and maple syrup to blend.
3. In a large bowl, combine the oats, coconut, salt, and cinnamon.

4. Add the warm liquid to the oat mixture and mix until fully incorporated.

5. Spread the mixture evenly on a cookie sheet and bake for for 8 to 10 hours. If the granola isn't crunchy enough, raise the temperature to 250°F to finish. If you raise the temperature, make sure to check frequently to keep the granola from burning. Remove from the oven and cool.

6. Add the toasted nuts and dried fruit and mix to incorporate. Store in an airtight container or freeze in bags.

NUTRITION FACTS

Serving Size: 2 oz ■ Servings Per Recipe: 8 ■ Amount Per Serving ■ Calories: 271 ■ Calories from fat: 83 (31% of tot cal) ■ % Daily Value* ■ Total Fat 9g 14% ■ Saturated Fat 3g 17% ■ Cholesterol 3mg 1% ■ Sodium 159mg 7% ■ Total Carbo 44g 15% ■ Dietary Fiber 5g 20% ■ Sugars 26g ■ Protein 5g ■ Vitamin A 8% ■ Vitamin C 1% ■ Calcium 3% ■ Iron 15%

*Percent Daily Values are based on a 2000 calorie diet. Your daily values may be higher or lower depending upon your caloric intake.

Johnny Cakes R

8 SERVINGS

When 4-year-old Ben Holmes tasted these, he leapt from his chair, jumped up and down and said, "I LOVE these, Mom!! I love the crusty part, it's really crunchy." His baby sister, Kaia, eats them all the time for snacks.

"I grew up in Hingham, Massachusetts, a small coastal town located just south of Boston, where Johnny Cakes are part of New England's rich culinary tradition. In nearby Little Compton, Rhode Island, at Sakonnet Vineyards Country Store, Susan and Earl Sampson serve Johnny Cakes for breakfast. I have made their Johnny Cakes a tradition in my life and I hope this recipe will become a tradition in your home."

— ANN COOPER

1½ cups cornmeal, yellow or white

1 cup all-purpose flour

½ cup sugar

1 teaspoon baking powder

1 teaspoon kosher salt

4 large eggs

1 cup + 2 tablespoons 1% milk

6 tablespoons (¾ stick) unsalted butter, melted

Maple syrup, jelly, jam, or fresh berries

1. In a medium bowl, combine the cornmeal, flour, sugar, baking powder, and salt and mix well.
2. In a small bowl, combine the eggs and milk. Whisk together until well blended. Add to the dry ingredients and mix well. Stir in the melted butter.
3. Preheat griddle till hot and grease.
4. Ladle approximately ¼ cup per cake onto the griddle. Flip when edges are firm and golden.
5. Serve with maple syrup, jellies, or jams, or with your favorite seasonal berry.

NUTRITION FACTS

Serving Size: 2 cakes ■ Servings Per Recipe: 8 ■ Amount Per Serving ■ Calories: 172 ■ Calories from fat: 60 (35% of tot cal) ■ % Daily Value* ■ Total Fat 7g 10% ■ Saturated Fat 4g 18% ■ Cholesterol 76mg 25% ■ Sodium 176mg 7% ■ Total Carbo 23g 8% ■ Dietary Fiber 1g 5% ■ Sugars 7g ■ Protein 4g ■ Vitamin A 33% ■ Vitamin C 0% ■ Calcium 4% ■ Iron 11%

*Percent Daily Values are based on a 2,000 calorie diet. Your daily values may be higher or lower depending upon your caloric intake.

 Despite USDA guidelines specifying that school lunches' fat content be 30 percent or less of total calories, school lunches average 34 percent.

Lemon-Ricotta Pancakes R

8 SERVINGS

One of the nice things about this recipe, besides the fact that it's delicious, is that adding the ricotta adds nutritional value without adding
fat. Pancakes are always a hit for breakfast and the flavor and texture of
these makes them a real favorite. The batter can also be used to make
incredible light, crispy waffles. Both pancakes and waffles are best eaten
right after they're cooked because they don't maintain their crispness
long after they come out of the pan or off the waffle iron. These pancakes are unbelievably good served as is, but if you want a topping we
recommend serving them with maple syrup or lemon marmalade. Fresh
strawberries complement the lemon flavor.

3 large eggs, separated

½ cup fat-free ricotta cheese, drained overnight if
    particularly wet

1 cup + 2 tablespoons 1% milk

½ cup buttermilk

1¾ cups all-purpose flour

1 tablespoon sugar

1 teaspoon baking powder

1 teaspoon baking soda

¼ teaspoon kosher salt

½ teaspoon lemon juice

½ teaspoon grated lemon zest

2 tablespoons canola oil for cooking

1. Put the egg yolks and ricotta in the bowl of a food processor or
   blender and process until smooth. Add the milk, buttermilk, flour,
   sugar, baking powder, baking soda, and salt, and continue to process

until everything is completely blended. Transfer to a large bowl.
Fold in the lemon juice and lemon zest.

2. Beat the egg whites in a medium bowl to soft peaks. Fold gently into
the batter.

3. Preheat and grease griddle. Ladle pancakes onto the griddle and
cook until golden brown. Flip when edges are firm and golden, then
cook other side until golden.

NUTRITION FACTS

Serving Size: 2 pancakes ■ Servings Per Recipe: 8 ■ Amount Per Serving ■ Calories: 195 ■ Calories
from fat: 59 (30% of tot cal) ■ % Daily Value* ■ Total Fat 7g 10% ■ Saturated Fat 1g 7% ■ Cholesterol
98mg 33% ■ Sodium 221mg 9% ■ Total Carbo 25g 8% ■ Dietary Fiber 1g 3% ■ Sugars 4g ■ Protein
8g ■ Vitamin A 17% ■ Vitamin C 1% ■ Calcium 6% ■ Iron 16%

*Percent Daily Values are based on a 2000 calorie diet. Your daily values may be higher or lower de-
pending upon your caloric intake.

Bread of the Dead CPF

16 SERVINGS

In Mexico one of the most revered holidays is the Day of the Dead
(November 1st). It is the day Mexicans remember their dead and celebrate the cycle of life. All over the country there are parades, festivi-
ties, prayers, and of course lots of eating. Shaped like people and
animals, and baked for both the living and the dead, Bread of the Dead
is a traditional holiday food. Kids will love making little dough people
and animals, so help them roll up their sleeves and get their hands in
the flour. Some of the most authentic Bread of the Dead recipes are
leavened with yeast, but this one is leavened with baking powder,
which shortens preparation time considerably. Store leftover bread in
an airtight container up to 2 or 3 days and put one in your child's lunch
box as a special treat.

2 cups + 1 tablespoon all-purpose flour

2 teaspoons baking powder

2 tablespoons granulated sugar

¼ teaspoon salt

1 egg

⅔ cup 2% milk

¼ cup vegetable oil

¼ cup light brown sugar, packed

1 teaspoon ground cinnamon

1 tablespoon unsalted butter, melted

1. Grease a large cookie sheet with oil and preheat oven to 350°F.
2. In a large bowl combine 2 cups flour, the baking powder, granulated sugar, and salt.
3. Stir in the egg, milk, and vegetable oil, mixing by hand until the dough comes together. Turn out onto a heavily floured surface and knead until the dough becomes smooth.
4. Mold bread into desired shapes and place on the prepared cookie sheet.
5. In a small bowl combine the brown sugar, 1 tablespoon flour, cinnamon, and melted butter and mix well. Sprinkle the cinnamon and sugar mixture on the tops of the bread shapes and bake for 20 to 25 minutes until golden.

NUTRITION FACTS

Serving Size: 1 piece ▪ Servings Per Recipe: 16 ▪ Amount Per Serving ▪ Calories: 126 ▪ Calories from fat: 45 (36% of tot cal) ▪ % Daily Value* ▪ Total Fat 5g 8% ▪ Saturated Fat 1g 5% ▪ Cholesterol 19mg 6% ▪ Sodium 101mg 4% ▪ Total Carbo 18g 6% ▪ Dietary Fiber 1g 2% ▪ Sugars 5g ▪ Protein 2g ▪ Vitamin A 6% ▪ Vitamin C 0% ▪ Calcium 7% ▪ Iron 10%

*Percent Daily Values are based on a 2000 calorie diet. Your daily values may be higher or lower depending upon your caloric intake.

 A 2003 government study of the school lunch program reported that 94 percent of high schools and 84 percent of middle schools sold soda or sugary fruit drinks in that year.

Sweet Potato Biscuits CPF

16 SERVINGS

Biscuits are a perfect snack. The addition of the sweet potatoes in this recipe adds flavor and nutrition—after all, sweet potatoes are a super-food, which means that they have a high nutrient-to-calorie ratio. These biscuits can also be served as part of a main meal. If you're out of sweet potatoes you can use any kind of sweet squash. Pumpkin (even canned if you're in a hurry) is a great substitute.

1½ cups all-purpose flour, plus extra for kneading
½ cup whole-wheat flour
1 tablespoon baking powder
1 teaspoon salt
4 tablespoons (½ stick) unsalted butter, cold
¾ cup milk
½ cup cooked and mashed sweet potatoes (1 large)

1. Preheat oven to 450°F.
2. Combine the flours, baking powder, and salt in a medium mixing bowl. Stir to mix well.
3. Cut the cold butter into small pieces and add to the flour mixture.
4. Using your fingertips, work the butter into the flour until it has the consistency of cornmeal.
5. In a small bowl, combine the milk and sweet potato and mix well using a fork or a whisk. Add to the flour mixture all at once and stir quickly just until it forms a ball.
6. Turn the dough out onto a lightly floured surface and knead 14 times. DO NOT overwork the dough or it will become tough.
7. Pat the dough out until it is ½ inch thick. Cut into rounds with a biscuit cutter or the floured top of a drinking glass.

8. Gather the scraps, pat out, and cut again until all the dough is used.

9. Place dough rounds on a cookie sheet and bake for 8 to 10 minutes, until the bottoms of the biscuits are golden brown.

NUTRITION FACTS

Serving Size: 1 biscuit ■ Servings Per Recipe: 16 ■ Amount Per Serving ■ Calories: 99 ■ Calories from fat: 31 (33% of tot cal) ■ % Daily Value* ■ Total Fat 3g 5% ■ Saturated Fat 2g 10% ■ Cholesterol 9mg 3% ■ Sodium 252mg 11% ■ Total Carbo 14g 5% ■ Dietary Fiber 1g 4% ■ Sugars 1g ■ Protein 2g ■ Vitamin A 187% ■ Vitamin C 4% ■ Calcium 9% ■ Iron 9%

*Percent Daily Values are based on a 2000 calorie diet. Your daily values may be higher or lower depending upon your caloric intake.

Potato-Chive Biscuits CPF

16 SERVINGS

Biscuits make a nice addition to a variety of meals. Try these as a topping for Chicken Pot Pie (page 168) or as a side with chicken or chili. Of course, they're great on their own as well and make for a tasty snack. Use 1-inch cutters to make snack-sized biscuits for small children and babies (and yes, babies will eat them!).

2 cups all-purpose flour, plus extra for the work surface

2 teaspoons baking powder

¼ teaspoon baking soda

1 teaspoon kosher salt

4 tablespoons (½ stick) unsalted butter, chilled

1 cup plain mashed potatoes (2 large)

¾ cup buttermilk

½ cup chopped chives

1. Preheat the oven to 450°F.

2. In a large bowl, combine the flour, baking powder, baking soda, and salt.

3. Cut the butter in small pieces and using your fingertips, rub the butter into the flour mixture until there are no lumps.

4. In another bowl, combine the mashed potatoes, buttermilk, and chives.

5. Pour the wet ingredients into the dry ingredients and mix until just combined.

6. Turn the dough out onto a floured surface and pat the dough out until it is ½-inch thick.

7. Cut the biscuits with a round cookie cutter or the floured top of a drinking glass and arrange on a cookie sheet. Gather up scraps and repeat until all the dough is used. Bake 10 to 15 minutes or until golden brown.

NUTRITION FACTS

Serving Size: 1 biscuit ■ Servings Per Recipe: 16 ■ Amount Per Serving ■ Calories: 99 ■ Calories from fat: 28 (28% of tot cal) ■ % Daily Value* ■ Total Fat 3g 5% ■ Saturated Fat 2g 9% ■ Cholesterol 8mg 3% ■ Sodium 255mg 11% ■ Total Carbo 15g 5% ■ Dietary Fiber 1g 3% ■ Sugars 1g ■ Protein 2g ■ Vitamin A 18% ■ Vitamin C 8% ■ Calcium 7% ■ Iron 9%

*Percent Daily Values are based on a 2000 calorie diet. Your daily values may be higher or lower depending upon your caloric intake.

Guacamole with Baked Tortilla Chips R

8 SERVINGS

Avocados are creamy, delicious, and very healthy—great as a snack, served with burritos, as a spread on any of the wrap sandwiches in this book, or as something different as part of lunch.

8 8-inch corn tortillas

2 very ripe Hass avocados

⅓ cup red onion (½ small), small diced

1 tablespoon jalapeño pepper (1 small), small diced

¼ cup Roma tomatoes (½ small), small diced

3 tablespoons chopped fresh cilantro

2 teaspoons lime juice

½ teaspoon kosher salt

⅛ teaspoon freshly ground black pepper

1. For the tortilla chips, preheat the oven to 350°F.
2. Cut tortillas into triangles, strips, or any shape your kids like. Spread on a cookie sheet in a single layer and bake until crisp, about 15 minutes.
3. Halve, pit, and scoop the avocados. Using a potato masher or a fork, mash them in a small bowl.
4. Mix in the onions, jalapeño, tomatoes, and cilantro.
5. Season with lime juice, salt, and pepper.

NUTRITION FACTS

Serving Size: ¼ cup dip plus 1 tortilla ■ Servings Per Recipe: 8 ■ Amount Per Serving ■ Calories: 132 ■ Calories from fat: 51 (39% of tot cal) ■ % Daily Value* ■ Total Fat 6g 9% ■ Saturated Fat 1g 4% ■ Cholesterol 0mg 0% ■ Sodium 233mg 10% ■ Total Carbo 18g 6% ■ Dietary Fiber 1g 5% ■ Sugars 0g ■ Protein 3g ■ Vitamin A 18% ■ Vitamin C 8% ■ Calcium 7% ■ Iron 10%

*Percent Daily Values are based on a 2,000 calorie diet. Your daily values may be higher or lower depending upon your caloric intake.

In 2005, vending machines serving up soda, candy and chips are in 58 percent of elementary schools, 84 percent of middle schools and 94 percent of high schools—with the profits often going to the school's general fund.

High-Protein Squares R

■

24 BARS

This snack makes a great replacement for processed "power" bars and they can be made ahead and kept in an airtight container for up to a week. If you can't find carob chips go ahead and substitute chocolate chips—the change in fat and calories is marginal. Organic chocolate chips are available in many supermarkets, so check those aisles first.

4 tablespoons (½ stick) butter

1¼ cups chunky peanut butter

1 cup carob chips

½ cup wheat germ

1 cup shredded unsweetened coconut

⅔ cup walnut pieces

¼ cup sesame seeds

¼ cup unsalted raw sunflower seeds

1. In a small saucepan over medium heat, melt together the butter, carob chips, and peanut butter.
2. In a medium bowl, combine all other ingredients. Drizzle with peanut butter mixture and mix well.
3. Press the mixture into an 8 × 12-inch pan. Chill until firm and cut into 24 squares.
4. To store, place in an airtight container in the refrigerator.

NUTRITION FACTS

Serving Size: One 2-inch square ■ Servings Per Recipe: 24 ■ Amount Per Serving ■ Calories: 132 ■ Calories from fat: 97 (73% of tot cal) ■ % Daily Value* ■ Total Fat 11g 17% ■ Saturated Fat 4g 17% ■ Cholesterol 5mg 2% ■ Sodium 53mg 2% ■ Total Carbo 7g 2% ■ Dietary Fiber 2g 7% ■ Sugars 4g ■ Protein 4g ■ Vitamin A 0% ■ Vitamin C 1% ■ Calcium 5% ■ Iron 9%

*Percent Daily Values are based on a 2000 calorie diet. Your daily values may be higher or lower depending upon your caloric intake.

Pizza Wheels R

16 SERVINGS

These pizza wheels are fast and easy to make, and the perfect size for a snack that won't interfere with dinner. Of course we prefer to see moms make the dough from scratch, but we know it's not always possible. Store-bought frozen bread and pizza doughs work great as well. Just check the ingredient list and make sure there aren't any artificial ingredients. Flour, salt, and yeast are about all you need to make a good dough and those are the ingredients you should see on the label.

2⅔ cups all-purpose flour, plus extra for kneading and
   rolling
⅔ teaspoon kosher salt
1½ teaspoons active dry yeast
1 cup warm 1% milk
2 tablespoons olive oil
¾ cup (6-ounce can) tomato paste
1 cup chopped onion (1 medium)
¾ cup chopped fresh pineapple
¾ cup chopped ham
1¼ cups (5 ounces) shredded sharp Cheddar cheese
⅓ cup chopped Italian flat-leaf parsley

1. Preheat the oven to 350°F.
2. Combine flour, salt, and yeast. Mix in warm milk and oil.
3. Knead for 10 minutes and then divide dough into two equal pieces.
4. Roll each piece out to a 12 × 8-inch rectangle and spread with tomato paste.
5. Combine onion, pineapple, ham, cheese, and parsley and sprinkle over the tomato paste.

6. Roll each rectangle lengthwise in jelly roll–style, cut into 16 slices each and bake for 25 minutes.

NUTRITION FACTS

Serving Size: 2 wheels ▪ Servings Per Recipe: 16 ▪ Amount Per Serving ▪ Calories: 162 ▪ Calories from fat: 55 (34% of tot cal) ▪ % Daily Value* ▪ Total Fat 6g 9% ▪ Saturated Fat 3g 13% ▪ Cholesterol 15mg 5% ▪ Sodium 331mg 14% ▪ Total Carbo 20g 7% ▪ Dietary Fiber 1g 5% ▪ Sugars 3g ▪ Protein 7g ▪ Vitamin A 45% ▪ Vitamin C 17% ▪ Calcium 10% ▪ Iron 15%

*Percent Daily Values are based on a 2000 calorie diet. Your daily values may be higher or lower depending upon your caloric intake.

Fruit Smoothie R

8 SERVINGS

Smoothies, the healthy alternative to milk shakes. As an after-school snack, these will be a big hit. They make a great breakfast beverage as well.

"Tracy-Lynn says, 'Fruitylicious!!!!!' This is coming from a smoothie specialist. She'd rather have a smoothie than anything!"

— LISA MACON, ORLANDO, FL, MOTHER OF TWO

3 ripe large bananas
1½ cups chopped fresh pineapple
1½ cups orange juice
1½ cups plain nonfat yogurt
16 to 18 ice cubes
¼ cup honey

Put all ingredients in batches in a blender and process until smooth. Serve.

NUTRITION FACTS

Serving Size: About 1 cup ■ Servings Per Recipe: 8 ■ Amount Per Serving ■ Calories: 105 ■ Calories from fat: 4 (4% of tot cal) ■ % Daily Value* ■ Total Fat 0g 0% ■ Saturated Fat 0g 1% ■ Cholesterol 1mg 0% ■ Sodium 37mg 2% ■ Total Carbo 24g 8% ■ Dietary Fiber 1g 4% ■ Sugars 20g ■ Protein 3g ■ Vitamin A 12% ■ Vitamin C 66% ■ Calcium 11% ■ Iron 3%

*Percent Daily Values are based on a 2,000 calorie diet. Your daily values may be higher or lower depending upon your caloric intake.

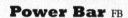

Power Bar FB

24 BARS

A lot of people rely on processed "power" bars for healthy snacks, but you can easily make them at home using whole ingredients. This bar was developed by FullBloom Baking Company for the Berkeley Unified School District. Whether your child plays sports or just needs a burst of energy to finish schoolwork, this bar is sure to please. Send one to school with a child who participates in after-school sports activities and will need extra energy late in the day.

⅓ cup canola oil, plus additional for the pan

½ cup honey

½ cup light corn syrup

2 cups rolled oats

3 cups puffed rice cereal

½ cup raisins

½ cup golden raisins

1½ cups almond pieces

¼ cup shredded unsweetened coconut

1. Preheat oven to 350°F. Grease a 9 × 12-inch pan.
2. Combine the oil, honey, and corn syrup and heat in the microwave on medium power until warm, approximately 1 minute.
3. In a large mixing bowl, combine the remaining ingredients. Toss together, and then pour the warm honey mixture over the dry ingredients. Mix to combine.
4. Pour the mixture into the prepared pan and spread evenly. Press down lightly. Bake for 15 minutes.
5. Allow to cool completely in the pan. Remove from the pan before cutting into 24 1½ × 3-inch bars. Store in an airtight container.

NUTRITION FACTS

Serving Size: One 1½ × 3-inch piece ■ Servings Per Recipe: 24 ■ Amount Per Serving ■ Calories: 159 ■ Calories from fat: 61 (38% of tot cal) ■ % Daily Value* ■ Total Fat 7g 10% ■ Saturated Fat 1g 4% ■ Cholesterol 0mg 0% ■ Sodium 10mg 0% ■ Total Carbo 24g 8% ■ Dietary Fiber 2g 7% ■ Sugars 16g ■ Protein 3g ■ Vitamin A 0% ■ Vitamin C 1% ■ Calcium 3% ■ Iron 13%

*Percent Daily Values are based on a 2000 calorie diet. Your daily values may be higher or lower depending upon your caloric intake.

Apple-Date Bars R

18 BARS

Afternoon snacks are an important part of every child's day, and recipes like this that incorporate fruit and nuts are nice to have on hand. These bars can be baked ahead, cut, and frozen in plastic bags and kept up to 2 months in the freezer. They even taste great right out of the freezer! Send one to school as a special treat every now and then.

"These are good, Mom! They taste like gingerbread men!"

— BEN HOLMES, FALMOUTH, MA, AGE 4

5 tablespoons butter, plus extra for the pan

2/3 cup (packed) brown sugar

1 large egg

3 tablespoons 2% milk

1/2 cup peeled and chopped apple (1 medium)

1 1/3 cups all-purpose flour

3/4 teaspoon baking soda

1/2 teaspoon ground cinnamon

1/4 teaspoon ground cloves

1/4 teaspoon ground nutmeg

1/2 cup walnut pieces

1/2 cup pitted and chopped dried dates

1. Preheat the oven to 350°F. Butter a 9 × 12-inch pan.
2. Cream the butter and brown sugar in a large mixing bowl. Mix in the egg and milk. Stir in the apple.
3. Add the flour, baking soda, cinnamon, cloves, and nutmeg, mix thoroughly. Stir in the nuts and dates.
4. Spread dough in the greased pan and bake for 20 to 25 minutes, until firm to the touch.
5. Remove from the oven and allow to cool for 10 minutes before cutting in 18 2 × 3-inch pieces.

NUTRITION FACTS

Serving Size: One 2 × 3-inch piece ■ Servings Per Recipe: 18 ■ Amount Per Serving ■ Calories: 136 ■ Calories from fat: 51 (38% of tot cal) ■ % Daily Value* ■ Total Fat 6g 9% ■ Saturated Fat 2g 11% ■ Cholesterol 22mg 7% ■ Sodium 88mg 4% ■ Total Carbo 20g 7% ■ Dietary Fiber 1g 4% ■ Sugars 11g ■ Protein 2g ■ Vitamin A 15% ■ Vitamin C 1% ■ Calcium 2% ■ Iron 8%

*Percent Daily Values are based on a 2000 calorie diet. Your daily values may be higher or lower depending upon your caloric intake.

Strawberries are the most pesticide-laden food of all. Because they're small and not easy to wash, choose organic ones to keep your family safe.

Quick Snacks

Chocolate–peanut butter bananas: Cut bananas in half widthwise, push a Popsicle stick in each half, spread liberally with peanut butter, dip in melted chocolate, and roll quickly in nuts. Freeze on a cookie sheet and then transfer to plastic freezer bags.

Yogurt dip: Mix yogurt with honey or jam and spices like nutmeg and cinnamon and serve with cut-up fruits on toothpicks.

Frozen grapes: Wash and bag them and throw them in the freezer for a great anytime snack.

Nuts: Nuts get a bad rap for their fat content, but they contain good fats and are a great source of protein. Expose your child to a large variety of nuts.

Dried fruits/organic fruit leathers: With their concentrated sweetness, they taste more like candy than something "healthy," and most kids love them. Usually one fruit leather is equal to one serving of fruit.

Fruit kebabs: Line bamboo skewers (trim off sharp tips for small children) with a variety of fruit—apple chunks, banana slices, grapes, and pieces of cantaloupe, pineapple, and watermelon. Kids love to help make these. Put them in the refrigerator where even small children can reach them. Serve alone or with yogurt dip (see above).

Popcorn: Rather than going for the microwave versions, many of which are loaded with trans fats, pop it the old-fashioned way. For great flavor, use olive oil and sprinkle with salt before popping. Looking for something different? Shake on some chili powder or even cinnamon and sugar. Let your kids come up with some healthy topping ideas as well.

Yogurt: Preportioned containers of organic yogurt are terrific snacks for kids.

Because we like to encourage kids to learn to make their own healthy choices, we're also big advocates of having fresh fruit and healthy snacks in places where children can reach them at all times. A fruit bowl filled with a variety of choices on the kitchen counter along with a "Healthy Snack Basket" works beautifully. Fill the snack basket with portable healthy snacks like fruit leathers, snack bars, preportioned bags of flavored popcorn or mixed nuts, or Granola (page 136).

Hummus R

24 SERVINGS

Once a novelty, hummus is now manufactured by dozens of companies and is available in grocery stores across the country. In a pinch you can buy it, but it's so easy to make you'll wonder why you ever bought it in the first place. We recommend using dried chickpeas for the most flavorful hummus, but if you don't have time, two cups of drained canned chick peas may be substituted for the dried beans in the recipe.

Hummus can be served as a main course or a snack. If you want to serve it as a snack we recommend baking pita triangles (350°F oven until crisp) to go with it.

    1 cup dried garbanzo beans (chickpeas)
    2 cups extra virgin olive oil
    1 tablespoon + 1½ teaspoons lemon juice
    3 cloves garlic
    3 tablespoons tahini
    ¼ teaspoon kosher salt
    ⅛ teaspoon freshly ground black pepper

1. In at least 4 cups of water, bring the garbanzo beans to a boil. Reduce to a simmer and cook until tender about 3 hours. Drain, but reserve some of the cooking liquid.

Conventionally produced raspberries often contain more than 39 chemicals; three of the pesticides found most often are captain, iprodione, and vinclozolin.

2. Combine all the ingredients in a food processor and process until very smooth. If the consistency is too thick, add some of the reserved cooking liquid and process again until smooth.

NUTRITION FACTS

Serving Size: 2 tablespoons ■ Servings Per Recipe: 24 ■ Amount Per Serving ■ Calories: 202 ■ Calories from fat: 176 (87% of tot cal) ■ % Daily Value* ■ Total Fat 20g 30% ■ Saturated Fat 3g 13% ■ Cholesterol 0mg 0% ■ Sodium 29mg 1% ■ Total Carbo 6g 2% ■ Dietary Fiber 2g 7% ■ Sugars 1g ■ Protein 2g ■ Vitamin A 1% ■ Vitamin C 2% ■ Calcium 2% ■ Iron 8%

*Percent Daily Values are based on a 2000 calorie diet. Your daily values may be higher or lower depending upon your caloric intake.

> **Never believe that a few caring people can't change the world . . . for indeed, that's all who ever have.**
>
> —MARGARET MEAD

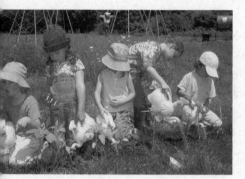

CHAPTER 5

Lunch

It will be wonderful when school lunches finally make the nutritional grade, but until then most of us will try to pack healthful lunches for our children to take to school. The recipes in this chapter will help you do that while adding variety and all sorts of new flavors to your child's diet.

In the interest of sustainability we encourage you to try cooking seasonally. In the fall in the northeastern United States, look for crisp apples, squashes, root vegetables, and dark, leafy greens like kale and Swiss chard. In winter, the focus will continue to be on the greens and root vegetables of fall, but it's also a great time to break out the bags of

Four- and five-year-old girls watering young sunflowers *Sarah Pring* dried legumes. They're a wonderful source of protein for your family, and as the weather grows cooler there is something about stewed beans that makes you feel like you're gearing up to cozy-in for the winter. Spring is the hardest time of year because it's too early for most fruits and vegetables. It does, however, bring us the first of the the season's greens. Asparagus is on its way, early spinach is tender and sweet, lettuces are growing, and so are fresh herbs like parsley, chives, sage, cilantro, and oregano. When we start considering spring recipes, they're usually a blend of the last of the late-winter harvest and the produce we're able to get at the beginning of the warm season. Of course, if you live in the warmer climates of California, Florida, Texas, and Arizona, not only does spring come earlier, but by April or May you'll see early peas, first of the season squash, and even some broccoli, broccoli rabe, and romanesco (a broccoli/cauliflower blend), not to mention strawberries and rhubarb.

In most states, kids are on break during the summer, which may take the focus off healthy eating because there are no lunches to pack and grabbing something on the run might be easier with a more hectic household. Don't let it be that way! Summer is the time to really get the family involved in cooking because there is no better time for fresh local produce. Everything is at its peak. Melons, berries, summer squashes, a huge variety of greens—and there is such a plethora, you can even get busy canning for the winter months. When you find your garden overrun by tomatoes and you can't eat your way out of your backyard, pick a huge bunch and start putting things up. Freeze berries and corn stripped from the cob. Peas and beans freeze beautifully as well. Make some jams and freeze a pie or two to have as a nice winter surprise. Get the kids in the kitchen or out on the back porch with you and give them each a job. They'll love shelling peas and husking corn. And get them out into your local berry patches to pick their own. They'll likely eat their weight in berries as they pick. If you don't have the time or space for your own garden, check around and see if you can get your kids involved in a summer gardening club like The Magic Garden Club (see page 109). You'll be amazed by how much they will enjoy planting and tending their own garden.

Pasta with Greens and Feta R

4 SERVINGS

This quick and easy pasta dish is both flavorful and flexible. Instead of spinach, greens could include arugula, watercress, or endive. For a more substantial meal, add roasted or grilled squash, eggplant, or peppers. It's easy to send to school, too, because pasta holds up well to dressings and moisture, and it tastes great at room temperature.

Salt
²⁄₃ pound penne pasta
1 cup diced yellow onion (1 medium)
2 tablespoons extra virgin olive oil
1 clove garlic, minced
2 cups washed and chopped fresh spinach
¼ cup water
2¼ teaspoons lemon juice
¼ teaspoon freshly ground black pepper
⅓ cup crumbled feta cheese

1. In a large pot of boiling salted water, cook the penne according to package directions until al dente. Drain and set aside.
2. In large sauté pan, sauté the onions in the oil until lightly browned. Add the garlic and cook for 2 minutes taking care not to burn. Add the spinach and water, cover the skillet and cook for 3 more minutes. When the spinach has wilted, add the pasta and toss to heat through.

Conventionally produced potatoes often contain more than 29 chemicals; the three pesticides most often found on potatoes are chlorpropham, thiabendazole, and endosulfans.

3. Add the lemon and pepper and toss again. Top with feta cheese and serve.

NUTRITION FACTS

Serving Size: About 5.5 ounces ■ Servings Per Recipe: 4 ■ Amount Per Serving ■ Calories: 391 ■ Calories from fat: 107 (27% of tot cal) ■ % Daily Value* ■ Total Fat 12g 18% ■ Saturated Fat 4g 20% ■ Cholesterol 17mg 6% ■ Sodium 229mg 10% ■ Total Carbo 60g 20% ■ Dietary Fiber 3g 12% ■ Sugars 3g ■ Protein 13g ■ Vitamin A 109% ■ Vitamin C 19% ■ Calcium 13% ■ Iron 7%

*Percent Daily Values are based on a 2000 calorie diet. Your daily values may be higher or lower depending upon your caloric intake.

Spinach and Black Bean Burritos with Salsa R

8 SERVINGS

Burritos make a great lunch box meal because they're self-contained—even more so than the average sandwich. For added protein serve them with rice and/or grated cheddar cheese. Although dry beans are best, organic, canned, low-fat refried beans would make a good substitute in the interest of time. For the lunch box, serve salsa on the side to avoid sogginess.

Burrito

1⅓ cups dried black beans

2½ teaspoons extra virgin olive oil

1 clove garlic, minced

¼ cup diced yellow onion (½ small)

1 teaspoon ground cumin

2½ teaspoons chopped fresh oregano

¾ teaspoon salt

3 tablespoons water

1 cup spinach, steamed and chopped (approx 1 pound)

8 6-inch flour tortillas

Salsa

2 cups diced canned plum tomatoes

2 tablespoons seeded and minced fresh jalapeño pepper (1 small)

2 tablespoons chopped fresh cilantro

1 clove garlic, minced

½ cup diced onion

4½ teaspoons lime juice

¾ teaspoon salt

1. In a large pot of water, simmer the black beans until tender. For about 4–6 hours quicker cooking, soak the beans in water overnight, drain the water, add fresh water and simmer for 1 to 2 hours. Drain and set aside.
2. In a medium mixing bowl combine all salsa ingredients, mix thoroughly, and set aside.
3. Heat the oil over medium heat in a medium-size sauté pan. Add the garlic and onion and sauté for 2 minutes.
3. Add the cumin, oregano, and salt, and cook for 1 minute.
4. Add the beans and water and cook for approximately 8 minutes. Remove from the heat and keep warm for assembly.
5. Assemble burritos by evenly distributing the spinach, beans, and salsa among the 8 tortillas. Roll up as desired and serve.

NUTRITION FACTS

Serving Size: 1 burrito ■ Servings Per Recipe: 8 ■ Amount Per Serving ■ Calories: 233 ■ Calories from fat: 46g (20% of tot cal) ■ % Daily Value* ■ Total Fat 5g 8% ■ Saturated Fat 1g 3% ■ Cholesterol 0mg 0% ■ Sodium 826mg 34% ■ Total Carbo 39g 13% ■ Dietary Fiber 6g 22% ■ Sugars 2g ■ Protein 10g ■ Vitamin A 551% ■ Vitamin C 74% ■ Calcium 24% ■ Iron 45%

*Percent Daily Values are based on a 2000 calorie diet. Your daily values may be higher or lower depending upon your caloric intake.

Laptop Lunches

The beginning of every school year brings a hunt for new lunch boxes. Since we want parents to stay as far away from processed, prepackaged foods as possible, we started looking around for a lunchbox that would allow parents to pack more wholesome lunches for their kids and we found the perfect one: The Laptop Lunch System.

Tammy Pelstring and Amy Hemmert, the creators of Laptop Lunches, met in 1995 at a new mothers' group when their children were just babies. They shared an interest in fitness and nutrition, and when their kids entered the public school system they were appalled by the heavily processed junk foods children were bringing to school in their lunch boxes. Not only were kids eating bad foods, but they were also generating tons of unrecoverable waste at every meal, so Tammy and Amy put their heads together, did some serious market research, and created Laptop Lunches, a system that helps parents put together "wholesome, low-waste lunches."

The basic Laptop Lunch system is a plastic lunchbox that holds five plastic containers (two small, two large—one of which is lidded—and one extra-small container for dip or a condiment) as well as a metal-and-plastic fork and spoon. In addition to the basic system, parents can purchase an insulated outer pack, a water bottle, wide-mouth vacuum bottles, and an ice pack.

We've field-tested this system and we absolutely love it! It's colorful and user-friendly and encourages healthy portioning. It's easy to clean, and kids love deciding what they'd like to have in each of the plastic containers. The insulated bag and ice pack keep foods cold for hours, and the water bottle is marked in 4-ounce increments, which we think is a great feature because it's easy to see just how much juice you're sending in your child's lunch (see Chef Ann's Healthy Kid's Meal Wheel, page 15, for portioning).

Best of all, unlike some of the other lunch boxes on the market, Laptop lunch boxes don't contain lead. To purchase or for information, visit www.laptop lunches.com.

Vegetable Lo Mein R

■

8 SERVINGS

Pasta is always a hit with kids and lo mein is no different. Teaching children to eat with chopsticks is great fun and opens the door to discussion of other cultures. Although many people believe Marco Polo discovered pasta in China and took it home to Italy, both cultures had their own form of pasta long before Polo's worldwide adventures. In Italian, pasta means "paste," in reference to the method of creating dough from flour, eggs, and water or milk. If you want to make this dish a main course by adding a protein, try tofu, chicken, or pork. It is an excellent choice for the lunch box because it can be eaten warm or at room temperature and extra marinating will only make the noodles more flavorful.

¾ pound lo mein noodles

Sesame oil (start with a small amount)

¼ cup hoisin sauce

2 tablespoons soy sauce

2 tablespoons canola oil

2 tablespoons minced fresh ginger

4½ teaspoons minced garlic (about 3 cloves)

⅓ cup sliced scallions (green onions)

1 cup julienned carrot (2 large)

1 cup thinly sliced celery (1–2 stalks)

1 cup thinly sliced red onion (1 medium)

¾ cup fresh bean sprouts

3 tablespoons chopped fresh cilantro

1. Cook the lo mein noodles in boiling salted water until al dente. Cool. Toss lightly with sesame oil to prevent sticking.

2. Combine the hoisin and soy sauces in a small bowl and mix well.

3. In a wok or a large skillet heat 1 tablespoon canola oil and quickly sauté the ginger, garlic, and scallions until they release aroma, then add the carrots, celery, and red onion and briefly sauté before adding the bean sprouts, about 2 minutes.

4. In a separate medium skillet, heat 1 tablespoon canola oil and sauté the noodles. When they are hot and look pan-fried or lightly browned, add them to the other sautéed ingredients in the large pan. Add the soy-hoisin mixture and stir to coat. Sprinkle with the chopped cilantro and serve.

NUTRITION FACTS

Serving Size: About 1 cup ■ Servings Per Recipe: 8 ■ Amount Per Serving ■ Calories: 188 ■ Calories from fat: 6 (3% of tot cal) ■ % Daily Value* ■ Total Fat 1g 1% ■ Saturated Fat 0g 1% ■ Cholesterol 0mg 0% ■ Sodium 739mg 31% ■ Total Carbo 41g 14% ■ Dietary Fiber 2g 7% ■ Sugars 3g ■ Protein 8g ■ Vitamin A 461% ■ Vitamin C 18% ■ Calcium 5% ■ Iron 18%

*Percent Daily Values are based on a 2000 calorie diet. Your daily values may be higher or lower depending upon your caloric intake.

Fresh Corn Soup FC

8 SERVINGS

As the old adage goes, a good growing season is one during which the "corn is knee-high by the Fourth of July." Corn is a culinary hallmark of late summer and early fall and this delicious soup highlights its natural sweet creaminess. If the flavor of cilantro is too strong for your liking, try replacing it with a mixture of Italian flat-leaf parsley and your favorite garden herbs. Sending this one to school is no problem—just get a good hot food thermos like the one at Laptop Lunches (www.laptop lunches.com). The Small Lunch Jar holds 2¼ cups and is perfect for soups, stews, and other foods that need to stay hot.

1 teaspoon olive oil

½ cup onion (½ medium), diced medium

1 teaspoon minced garlic (1 clove)

½ teaspoon ground cumin

4 cups fresh corn kernels (2 to 3 ears)

2½ cups unpeeled red potatoes (2 large), diced medium

½ teaspoon kosher salt

⅛ teaspoon freshly ground black pepper

1 quart vegetable stock

¾ cup 1% milk

1 teaspoon chopped cilantro

1. Heat the oil in a 6- or 8-quart stockpot and sauté onions, garlic, and cumin over medium heat for 5 minutes or until the onions are translucent.

2. Add the corn, potatoes, salt, pepper, and stock. Bring to a boil. Reduce to a simmer and cook for 20 minutes or until the potatoes are soft.

3. Add the milk and cilantro and stir to heat through.

Serve with a garden-fresh salad.

NUTRITION FACTS

Servings Size: About 1 cup ■ Servings Per Recipe: 8 ■ Amount Per Serving ■ Calories: 137 ■ Calories from fat: 21 (15% of tot cal) ■ % Daily Value* ■ Total Fat 2g 4% ■ Saturated Fat 1g 3% ■ Cholesterol 3mg 1% ■ Sodium 440mg 18% ■ Total Carbo 28g 9% ■ Dietary Fiber 3g 14% ■ Sugars 5g ■ Protein 5g ■ Vitamin A 28% ■ Vitamin C 24% ■ Calcium 4% ■ Iron 10%

*Percent Daily Values are based on a 2000 calorie diet. Your daily values may be higher or lower depending upon your caloric intake.

 At a time when we need more exercise, walking declined by more than half between 1980 and 2000.

Harvest Hash FC

■

8 SERVINGS

This hearty hash can be a wonderful part of a Sunday brunch—served with eggs or as a side dish for chicken or pork. In late fall/early winter months, try replacing the butternut squash with your favorite variety of winter squash from your local farm stand or farmers' market.

1 teaspoon minced garlic (1 clove)

1 cup onion (1 medium), diced medium

2 tablespoons unsalted butter

1 tablespoon extra virgin olive oil

1¼ cups rutabaga (1 large), diced large

1¼ cups unpeeled red potatoes (1 large), diced large

1¼ cups butternut squash, peeled (1 large), diced large

1¼ cups parsnips, peeled (2 to 3), diced large

¾ teaspoon kosher salt

⅛ teaspoon freshly ground black pepper

½ teaspoon freshly ground nutmeg

1 teaspoon chopped fresh sage

4 tablespoons vegetable stock

1. In a large skillet with a cover, sauté the garlic and onions in the butter and oil until the onions are lightly browned.
2. Add the rutabaga, potatoes, squash, and parsnips and sauté for five minutes.

In 1970 there were 70,000 fast-food restaurants in our country; in 2001, there were more than 186,000.

3. Add the salt, pepper, nutmeg, and sage and stir to combine. Add the stock and mix well. Cover and simmer for 10 minutes or until the vegetables are tender. Serve.

NUTRITION FACTS

Serving Size: About 1 cup ■ Servings Per Recipe: 8 ■ Amount Per Serving ■ Calories: 108 ■ Calories from fat: 60 (55% of tot cal) ■ % Daily Value* ■ Total Fat 7g 10% ■ Saturated Fat 2g 12% ■ Cholesterol 8mg 3% ■ Sodium 327mg 14% ■ Total Carbo 11g 4% ■ Dietary Fiber 3g 11% ■ Sugars 3g ■ Protein 1g ■ Vitamin A 29% ■ Vitamin C 33% ■ Calcium 3% ■ Iron 7%

*Percent Daily Values are based on a 2000 calorie diet. Your daily values may be higher or lower depending upon your caloric intake.

Kale and White-Bean Soup FC

8 SERVINGS

Calcium is very much in the news these days. Indeed, parents should take heed. Research shows that girls have all the calcium their bones will absorb by the time they are 20 to 25 years old. After that, calcium stores are depleted, so it makes good sense to get it into your children's diets whenever possible. This soup has two great sources of calcium—kale and beans—so besides being delicious, it's also a great way to add calcium to your family's diet.

In 1968, McDonald's operated about 1,000 restaurants; today, there are about 31,000 worldwide, of which approximately 14,000 are in this country.

½ pound (about 1 cup) dried cannellini beans

1½ cups diced onion (1½ medium)

1½ tablespoons extra virgin olive oil

½ teaspoon minced garlic (½ clove)

1 quart vegetable stock (plus a bit more to adjust liquid to taste)

1 teaspoon kosher salt

⅛ teaspoon freshly ground black pepper

1 bay leaf

½ teaspoon roughly chopped fresh rosemary

2 cups carrots (4 large), diced medium

7 cups chopped kale (2 to 3 bunches)

¾ cup grated Parmesan cheese

1. Cook the beans in a large pot of boiling water until tender, about 1 to 1½ hours. Drain and set aside. You should have about 2½ cups.

2. In a 6- or 8-quart stockpot, sauté the onions in the oil for 5 minutes or until soft. Add the garlic and cook for an additional minute.

3. Add the cooked beans, stock, salt, pepper, bay leaf, and rosemary and simmer for 10 minutes.

4. Add the carrots and cook another 5 minutes.

5. Add the kale and cook about 12 minutes or until kale is tender. Add more vegetable stock if your soup needs more liquid, and warm through.

6. Check seasoning, adjust as needed, and remove the bay leaf. Serve sprinkled with grated Parmesan.

NUTRITION FACTS

Serving Size: About 1 cup ■ Servings Per Recipe: 8 ■ Amount Per Serving ■ Calories: 203 ■ Calories from fat: 50 (25% of tot cal) ■ % Daily Value* ■ Total Fat 6g 9% ■ Saturated Fat 2g 10% ■ Cholesterol 6mg 2% ■ Sodium 639mg 27% ■ Total Carbo 29g 10% ■ Dietary Fiber 10g 38% ■ Sugars 3g ■ Protein 11g ■ Vitamin A 1431% ■ Vitamin C 139% ■ Calcium 26% ■ Iron 33%

*Percent Daily Values are based on a 2000 calorie diet. Your daily values may be higher or lower depending upon your caloric intake.

Orzo Salad CPF

8 SERVINGS

Orzo is a nice little pasta that is great in salads and side dishes. We love the fresh flavors of the herbs and lemon juice. Enlist your children to help you experiment with different herbs and vegetables by asking them to come up with some of their favorite combinations. Send this to school as a side dish to a wrap sandwich. If you want to enhance the nutritional value of this salad, use whole-wheat orzo.

1 pound orzo pasta

5 tablespoons chopped fresh oregano

5 tablespoons chopped fresh mint leaves

6 tablespoons olive oil

3 tablespoons fresh lemon juice

½ teaspoon kosher salt

Freshly ground black pepper

1. Cook orzo in boiling water until tender, drain, and put in a large mixing bowl. Add oregano and mint and toss to combine.
2. In a small bowl combine the oil and lemon juice and add to orzo mixture, mixing well.
3. Season with salt and pepper to taste.

NUTRITION FACTS

Serving Size: About ½ cup ■ Servings Per Recipe: 8 ■ Amount Per Serving ■ Calories: 175 ■ Calories from fat: 103 (59% of tot cal) ■ % Daily Value* ■ Total Fat 11g 17% ■ Saturated Fat 2g 8% ■ Cholesterol 23mg 8% ■ Sodium 196mg 8% ■ Total Carbo 16g 5% ■ Dietary Fiber 2g 6% ■ Sugars 0g ■ Protein 3g ■ Vitamin A 39% ■ Vitamin C 10% ■ Calcium 7% ■ Iron 25%

*Percent Daily Values are based on a 2000 calorie diet. Your daily values may be higher or lower depending upon your caloric intake.

Chicken Pot Pie R

■

8 SERVINGS

Savory pot pies are fall favorites in New England, and this recipe was a particular favorite of the students at the Ross School in New York. You can make this a day ahead—it tastes even better after a night in the refrigerator. It's simple to prepare, but if you know you're going to be short on time it's best to put it all together the night before—minus the biscuits, of course, which are tastiest hot out of the oven. If you're sending this to school, put it in a wide-mouth vacuum bottle and serve the biscuit on the side.

2 cups onion (2 medium), diced medium

½ cup celery (1 stalk), diced medium

3 tablespoons unsalted butter

1 cup carrots (2 large), diced medium

2 cups potatoes (2 large), diced medium

1½ pounds boneless skinless chicken breasts, diced large

2 tablespoons all-purpose flour

2 bay leaves

3¾ cups 1% milk

3¾ cups chicken stock

1 tablespoon chopped fresh tarragon

1 tablespoon chopped fresh parsley

1 teaspoon kosher salt

⅛ teaspoon freshly ground black pepper

4 Potato-Chive or Sweet Potato Biscuits (pages 142 and 143),
   cut in half

1. Preheat oven to 400°F.
2. In a large pot, sauté the onions and celery in the butter until the

onions are translucent, about 2 minutes. Add the carrots and potatoes and cook until the hard vegetables are soft, about 4 minutes.

3. Add the chicken and cook for 3 minutes.

4. Stir in the flour and cook 3 minutes.

5. Add the bay leaves, milk, and chicken stock and cook until the vegetables are tender, about 5 minutes

6. Stir in the tarragon and parsley, season with salt and pepper, and
cook for 5 minutes until the flavors are blended and the chicken is
fully cooked.

8. To serve, place in individual bowls and top with half a biscuit.

NUTRITION FACTS

Serving Size: About 2 cups ■ Servings Per Recipe: 8 ■ Amount Per Serving ■ Calories: 380 ■ Calories
from fat: 116 (31% of tot cal) ■ % Daily Value* ■ Total Fat 13g 20% ■ Saturated Fat 6g 32% ■ Cholesterol 125mg 42% ■ Sodium 1516mg 63% ■ Total Carbo 28g 9% ■ Dietary Fiber 3g 14% ■ Sugars 10g
■ Protein 37g ■ Vitamin A 839% ■ Vitamin C 45% ■ Calcium 22% ■ Iron 25%

*Percent Daily Values are based on a 2000 calorie diet. Your daily values may be higher or lower de-
pending upon your caloric intake.

Note: Biscuits not included in Nutrition Facts

Pumpkin Curry CPF

8 SERVINGS

This recipe combines the glorious and intriguing flavors of the Far East
with the commonplace pumpkin. Dried curry powder evokes the flavors of India and coconut milk is reminiscent of the red, yellow, and
green curries of Thailand. This unusual and flavorful curry is a delight
that kids seem to love. If you're sending this to school, undercook the
rice a bit, mix it with the hot curry, and pack it in a wide-mouth vacuum bottle.

2 cups dry chick peas (garbanzo beans)

2 tablespoons olive oil

3 cups fresh pumpkin, peeled and diced

1 medium onion, peeled and diced

2 cups washed and roughly chopped kale

2 tablespoons curry powder

2 cups coconut milk

6 cups vegetable stock

1/2 teaspoon salt

Freshly ground black pepper to taste

Cooked rice, preferably brown

1. *The night before:* Soak the chick peas in water in a medium saucepan.
2. *The next day:* Cook the chick peas in water until soft, approximately 2½ hours at a simmer. Drain and set aside.
3. Heat the olive oil in a large pot and add the pumpkin, onion, kale, and curry powder. Sauté 10 minutes or until the pumpkin is tender.
4. Add the chick peas, coconut milk, vegetable stock, salt, and pepper.
5. Simmer 5 minutes.
6. Serve with rice.

NUTRITION FACTS

Serving Size: About 2 cups ▪ Servings Per Recipe: 8 ▪ Amount Per Serving ▪ Calories: 386 ▪ Calories from fat: 190 (49% of tot cal) ▪ % Daily Value* ▪ Total Fat 21g 32% ▪ Saturated Fat 14g 68% ▪ Cholesterol 0mg 0% ▪ Sodium 425mg 18% ▪ Total Carbo 42g 14% ▪ Dietary Fiber 11g 46% ▪ Sugars 10g ▪ Protein 12g ▪ Vitamin A 232% ▪ Vitamin C 67% ▪ Calcium 12% ▪ Iron 53%

*Percent Daily Values are based on a 2000 calorie diet. Your daily values may be higher or lower depending upon your caloric intake.

Note: Rice not included in Nutrition Facts.

 In 1970, Americans spent $6.2 billion on fast food; in 2004, they spent $124 billion.

Carrot-Ginger Soup R

8 SERVINGS

Soup makes for a tasty lunch at home or in a wide-mouthed vacuum bottle for school. The blend of Asian flavors and citrus in this recipe are pleasantly refreshing additions. A few tips: Ginger can be easily peeled with a spoon—just scrape the skin away. It's much faster and you'll have a lot less waste. If you're making fresh vegetable stock, take time to make a double or triple batch, use what you need, and freeze the rest in ice-cube trays or quart containers. Store the stock cubes in plastic freezer bags and use them as needed. This method works for all stocks.

1 teaspoon peeled and grated fresh ginger
½ cup leek (½ leek), ¼-inch slices
1 tablespoon canola oil
1 quart vegetable stock
1 tablespoon + 1 teaspoon soy sauce
1 teaspoon salt
¼ teaspoon freshly ground black pepper
2½ cups carrots (3 to 4 large), diced large
1 cup celery (1 to 2 stalks), diced large
1 tablespoon orange juice

1. In a large saucepan, sauté the ginger and leeks in canola oil until tender.
2. Add the stock, soy sauce, salt, and pepper. Bring to a boil and reduce to simmer for 10 minutes.
3. Add carrots and celery and cook for 20 minutes. Remove from heat and purée with a hand blender or in a standard blender.
4. Add the orange juice, check seasoning, and serve.

NUTRITION FACTS
Serving Size: About 1 cup ■ Servings Per Recipe: 8 ■ Amount Per Serving ■ Calories: 45 ■ Calories from fat: 17 (38% of tot cal) ■ % Daily Value* ■ Total Fat 2g 3% ■ Saturated Fat 0g 1% ■ Cholesterol 0mg 0% ■ Sodium 708mg 29% ■ Total Carbo 6g 2% ■ Dietary Fiber 2g 6% ■ Sugars 3g ■ Protein 1g ■ Vitamin A 1128% ■ Vitamin C 14% ■ Calcium 2% Iron 5%

*Percent Daily Values are based on a 2000 calorie diet. Your daily values may be higher or lower depending upon your caloric intake.

Autumn Harvest Soup CPF

8 SERVINGS

This soup showcases the sweetness of squash, making it an instant hit with kids. The Swiss chard adds valuable nutrition and calcium and the bulgur adds a nutty heartiness.

"This soup was so good, I can't wait to make it again!"

— ALICE LEGARDE, KINGWOOD, TX, MOTHER OF THREE,
GRANDMOTHER OF FIVE

4 tablespoons olive oil

2 leeks, white part only, thinly sliced

3 large carrots, peeled and chopped

3 stalks celery, chopped

3 cups fresh pumpkin, peeled and cubed

3 cups assorted squash such as butternut, buttercup, acorn, turban,
    peeled and cubed

5 sprigs fresh thyme

3 cloves garlic, minced

3 tablespoons minced fresh parsley

1 quart vegetable stock

¾ cup bulgur wheat, soaked in water until tender and drained

1 bunch Swiss chard, coarsely chopped (leaves and tender stems)

5 medium tomatoes, diced small

Salt

Freshly ground black pepper

1. Heat the oil in a large stockpot and sauté the leeks, carrots, and celery for 5 minutes.
2. Add the pumpkin, squash, thyme, garlic, and parsley. Stir in the stock and bring to a simmer. Cook for 10 to 15 minutes or until the pumpkin and squash are tender.
3. Add the bulgur, chard, and tomatoes and simmer another 10 minutes.
4. Season with salt and pepper and serve.

NUTRITION FACTS

Serving Size: 2 cups ▪ Servings Per Recipe: 8 ▪ Amount Per Serving ▪ Calories: 220 ▪ Calories from fat: 70 (32% of tot cal) ▪ % Daily Value* ▪ Total Fat 8g 12% ▪ Saturated Fat 1g 5% ▪ Cholesterol 0mg 0% ▪ Sodium 364mg 15% ▪ Total Carbo 36g 12% ▪ Dietary Fiber 9g 34% ▪ Sugars 6g ▪ Protein 6g ▪ Vitamin A 2255% ▪ Vitamin C 145% ▪ Calcium 14% ▪ Iron 43%

*Percent Daily Values are based on a 2000 calorie diet. Your daily values may be higher or lower depending upon your caloric intake.

Mediterranean Chicken Wrap R

8 SERVINGS

Wraps are a great way to make a sandwich that won't fall apart, and some kids actually prefer wraps to traditional between-the-bread sandwiches. All kinds of variations are possible with this one—try it with olives, tapenade, grilled zucchini, eggplant, or summer squash.

8 6-inch flour tortillas

½ cup Basil Pesto (below)

1¼ pounds roast chicken (meat only), shredded

1½ cups portabella mushrooms (2 large), roasted and sliced

1 cup red bell peppers (2 medium), roasted, peeled, and sliced

1 small red onion, thinly sliced

1 head Boston lettuce, shredded

¼ teaspoon salt

⅛ teaspoon freshly ground black pepper

On each of the tortillas place basil pesto, chicken, roasted mushrooms and peppers, onion, lettuce, and seasonings. Fold in ends and roll.

NUTRITION FACTS

Serving Size: 1 wrap ▪ Servings Per Recipe: 8 ▪ Amount Per Serving ▪ Calories: 288 ▪ Calories from fat: 118 (41% of tot cal) ▪ % Daily Value* ▪ Total Fat 9g 14% ▪ Saturated Fat 2g 10% ▪ Cholesterol 49mg 16% ▪ Sodium 409mg 17% ▪ Total Carbo 30g ▪ Dietary Fiber 1g 4% ▪ Sugars 3g ▪ Protein 22g ▪ Vitamin A 145% ▪ Vitamin C 90% ▪ Calcium 16% Iron 21%

*Percent Daily Values are based on a 2000 calorie diet. Your daily values may be higher or lower depending upon your caloric intake.

Basil Pesto R

2 CUPS

Pesto is one of the most all-purpose sauces in the kitchen. It can be used as a topping for pasta, a dressing for pasta salad, a marinade for grilled chicken or pork, and even a sandwich spread. And basil isn't the only herb that can be used—it can be made with sage, arugula, and a wide variety of other green herbs and vegetables.

2 cups fresh basil, chopped

6 tablespoons pine nuts, toasted and cooled

1 clove garlic, sliced

1 cup extra virgin olive oil

¼ cup grated Parmesan cheese

1. Put the basil, pine nuts, and garlic in the bowl of a food processor and pulse until fairly smooth.
2. Pour three-quarters of the olive oil into running food processor in a steady stream until the mixture is thick but liquid.
3. Add the Parmesan and continue to process. Adjust to the desired consistency with the remaining oil. Check seasoning and adjust if necessary. Use immediately or cover with a thin layer of olive oil and store in the refrigerator.

NUTRITION FACTS

Serving Size: 1 tablespoon ■ Servings Per Recipe: 32 ■ Amount Per Serving ■ Calories: 50 ■ Calories from fat: 48 (60% of tot cal) ■ % Daily Value* ■ Total Fat 5g 8% ■ Saturated Fat 1g 7% ■ Cholesterol 1mg 0% ■ Sodium 19mg 1% ■ Total Carbo 0g 0% ■ Dietary Fiber 0g 1% ■ Sugars 0g ■ Protein 1g ■ Vitamin A 23% ■ Vitamin C 2% ■ Calcium 4% ■ Iron 4%

*Percent Daily Values are based on a 2000 calorie diet. Your daily values may be higher or lower depending upon your caloric intake.

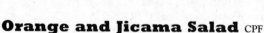

Orange and Jicama Salad CPF

8 SERVINGS

Citrus is synonymous with winter in California. Over the years Ann has come to love the plethora of citrus available in northern California, from Meyer lemons to heirloom limes and grapefruit—the flavors often astound. This recipe pairs the shining flavors of fresh citrus with the crunch and sweetness of jicama and the bite of jalapeño and cilantro. It makes a lovely side dish for sandwiches and burritos, and satisfies the urge many of us have for something crunchy with a sandwich.

> 6 medium navel oranges
> 1 medium jicama
> 5 sprigs cilantro
> 1 teaspoon minced jalapeño pepper
> Juice of 1 lime (1 to 2 tablespoons)
> Salt

1. Peel the oranges, taking care to remove pith, and jicama with a paring knife and cut into small pieces.
2. Pick the leaves off the cilantro sprigs and discard the stems. Roughly chop the leaves.
3. Combine the oranges, jicama, jalapeño, and cilantro in a medium bowl.
4. Add the lime juice and salt to taste, mix well, and let marinate for one hour before serving at room temperature

NUTRITION FACTS

Serving Size: About ¾ cup ■ Servings Per Recipe: 8 ■ Amount Per Serving ■ Calories: 84 ■ Calories from fat: 2 (2% of tot cal) ■ % Daily Value* ■ Total Fat 0g 0% ■ Saturated Fat 0g 0% ■ Cholesterol 0mg 0% ■ Sodium 51mg 2% ■ Total Carbo 21g 6% ■ Dietary Fiber 6g 23% ■ Sugars 14g ■ Protein 2g ■ Vitamin A 35% ■ Vitamin C 191% ■ Calcium 7% ■ Iron 5%

*Percent Daily Values are based on a 2000 calorie diet. Your daily values may be higher or lower depending upon your caloric intake.

 Harvard Medical School nutritionists report that "by our most conservative estimate, replacement of partially hydrogenated fat in the US diet with natural unhydrogenated vegetable oils would prevent between 30,000 and 100,000 premature deaths a year."

Grilled Beef Salad with Tatsoi R

■

8 SERVINGS

We don't advocate eating beef too often, both because it's not good for the planet and because beef is higher in fat than most other meats. But every once in a while it can be a real treat. This Asian-influenced salad is great on its own or even wrapped in a tortilla for the lunch box. Remember to cut the meat against the grain.

¼ teaspoon minced ginger

¼ teaspoon minced garlic

1 tablespoon + 1½ teaspoons Chinese mustard seeds

¼ teaspoon Chinese chili powder

2 tablespoons + 1½ teaspoons soy sauce

2 tablespoons + 1½ teaspoons water

2 tablespoons lime juice

1 tablespoon fish sauce

1 cup vegetable oil

2 pounds flank steak

1 cup thinly sliced red onion (1 medium)

4 cups tatsoi (Japanese mustard greens)

½ cup julienned radishes

1. In a medium bowl combine the ginger, garlic, mustard seeds, chili powder, soy sauce, water, lime juice, and fish sauce. Stir to mix, and while whisking constantly slowly add the oil in a thin stream until the dressing emulsifies, or comes together so that there is no separation of oil and the other liquids.
2. In an glass baking dish, marinate the flank steak in some of the dressing for 1 or 2 hours.

3. While the meat is marinating, prepare the grill, then grill the beef until medium rare and set aside to cool. Discard the marinade. When fully cooled, slice the meat in thin (¼-inch) slices against the grain.

4. Whisk the remaining dressing to recombine. In a large bowl, combine the onions, tatsoi, and radishes and toss with the dressing. Top the salad with sliced beef and serve.

NUTRITION FACTS

Serving Size: 1 cup ■ Servings Per Recipe: 8 ■ Amount Per Serving ■ Calories: 455 ■ Calories from fat: 328 (72% of tot cal) ■ % Daily Value* ■ Total Fat 36g 56% ■ Saturated Fat 6g 28% ■ Cholesterol 57mg 19% ■ Sodium 592mg 25% ■ Total Carbo 7g 2% ■ Dietary Fiber 2g 8% ■ Sugars 3g ■ Protein 26g ■ Vitamin A 89% ■ Vitamin C 39% ■ Calcium 10% ■ Iron 33%

*Percent Daily Values are based on a 2000 calorie diet. Your daily values may be higher or lower depending upon your caloric intake.

Brown Rice and Tofu Salad R

8 SERVINGS

This is a wonderful way to add a whole grain into your child's diet. The tofu adds protein, and the flavors complement each other beautifully. Serve it as a side dish in a boxed lunch or add grilled chicken or shrimp to make an entrée.

6 tablespoons + 1½ teaspoons soy sauce

2 teaspoons minced fresh ginger

2 tablespoons canola oil

¼ teaspoon crushed red pepper flakes

1 teaspoon rice syrup or honey

¾ teaspoon sesame oil

½ pound firm tofu in one piece

4 cups water

1 cup brown rice

½ cup thinly sliced scallions (green onions) (2 to 3 stalks)

1. In a small bowl, combine the soy sauce, ginger, canola oil, ⅛ teaspoon of the red pepper flakes, rice syrup, and sesame oil to make the marinade.

2. Add the tofu, turn gently to coat, and marinate overnight.

3. The next day, place the tofu in a colander set in a large bowl in the refrigerator. Press the tofu under about 1 pound of weight and drain for at least 4 hours. Reserve the marinade in the bowl.

4. While the tofu is draining, bring the water to a boil. Add the rice and cook until al dente, about 45 minutes. Drain and spread it on a cookie sheet to cool.

5. Remove the tofu from the colander and cut into bite-sized pieces (½-inch cubes). Put back into the bowl with the marinade. Add the cooled rice and toss gently to combine.

6. Add the scallions and remaining ⅛ teaspoon red pepper flakes, and mix gently. Taste and adjust seasoning if necessary.

NUTRITION FACTS

Serving Size: ½ cup ■ Servings Per Recipe: 8 ■ Amount Per Serving ■ Calories: 148 ■ Calories from fat: 47 (32% of tot cal) ■ % Daily Value* ■ Total Fat 5g 8% ■ Saturated Fat 1g 3% ■ Cholesterol 0mg 0% ■ Sodium 671mg 28% ■ Total Carbo 20g 7% ■ Dietary Fiber 1g 4% ■ Sugars 1g ■ Protein 5g ■ Vitamin A 5% ■ Vitamin C 3% ■ Calcium 3% Iron 11%

*Percent Daily Values are based on a 2000 calorie diet. Your daily values may be higher or lower depending upon your caloric intake.

 The USDA says that Americans eat 1 million animals an hour—mostly chickens but also cows, pigs, lambs, and others.

Vegetarian Black Bean Chili R

8 SERVINGS

For the bone-chilling days of winter, this is a terrific warming lunch for home or school. Squash, eggplant, and even greens can be added for different flavors. Not a fan of seitan? Replace it with extra firm tofu or ground turkey if you want a nonvegetarian version. Soak the beans overnight to shorten the overall cooking time. If you're sending it to school, the best way is in a wide-mouthed vacuum bottle.

1½ cups black beans, sorted, soaked, and drained

3 bay leaves

2¼ cups Spanish onion (2 medium), diced

3 cloves garlic, chopped

1 teaspoon canola oil

1½ teaspoons toasted and ground ancho chile

1½ teaspoons toasted and ground chipotle chile

1½ teaspoons toasted and ground whole cumin seed

¾ teaspoon kosher salt

¼ teaspoon freshly ground black pepper

½ cup crumbled seitan

⅓ cup green bell pepper (1 small), diced

¾ cup red bell pepper (1 medium), diced

¾ cup fresh Roma tomatoes (2 to 3), peeled, seeded, and chopped

1 tablespoon chopped cilantro

1. Cook the beans and the bay leaves in a large saucepan with water several inches above the top of the beans, until tender. Drain and reserve the cooking liquid. Discard the bay leaves.

2. Sauté the onions and garlic in the oil in another large saucepan until translucent.

3. Add the chiles, cumin, salt, and pepper and stir.
4. Add the seitan and cook for 5 minutes.
5. Add the peppers and continue cooking until peppers begin to soften, about 2 minutes, then add the tomatoes, beans, and enough cooking liquid to bring the mixture to the consistency of chili. Heat until hot.
6. Check and adjust seasoning one last time and stir in fresh cilantro. Serve.

NUTRITION FACTS

Serving Size: 1 cup ■ Servings Per Recipe: 8 ■ Amount Per Serving ■ Calories: 91 ■ Calories from fat: 10g 11% ■ % Daily Value* ■ Total Fat 1g 2% ■ Saturated Fat 0g 1% ■ Cholesterol 0mg 0% ■ Sodium 163mg 7% ■ Total Carbo 16g 5% ■ Dietary Fiber 5g 18% ■ Sugars 3g ■ Protein 6g ■ Vitamin A 122% ■ Vitamin C 89% ■ Calcium 4 % ■ Iron 16%

*Percent Daily Values are based on a 2000 calorie diet. Your daily values may be higher or lower depending upon your caloric intake.

Hearty Rutabaga Soup FC

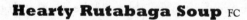

8 SERVINGS

Root vegetables are so much a part of our winter pantry here in the Northeast. The Ross School purchased literally tons of them and served them from December until March or April. This hearty soup will warm the chills of fall and winter right out of your family and travels well packed in a vacuum bottle for lunch at school.

Today Americans spend 90 percent of their food budget on processed foods.

2½ cups peeled rutabaga (1 large), diced large

3½ cups chopped carrots (4 large)

1½ cups peeled golden turnips (1 medium), diced large

1½ cups peeled parsnips (2), diced large

4½ teaspoons olive oil

1 cup onion (1 medium), diced medium

3 tablespoons unsalted butter

1½ teaspoons brown sugar

½ teaspoon finely chopped fresh rosemary

4 cups vegetable stock

1 teaspoon salt

⅛ teaspoon freshly ground black pepper

1. Preheat the oven to 350°F. Coat rutabaga, carrots, turnips, and parsnips in olive oil and roast on a cookie sheet for approximately 20 minutes until tender and slightly caramelized.

2. In a large saucepan, sauté onion in butter until soft. Add the brown sugar and cook 2 minutes.

3. Add the rosemary and cook 1 minute, then add the stock, and bring to a boil.

4. Add the roasted vegetables and bring to boil before reducing to a simmer for 10 minutes.

5. Puree until smooth with a handheld blender and add the salt and pepper, adjusting as needed.

NUTRITION FACTS

Serving Size: 1½ cups ■ Servings Per Recipe: 8 ■ Amount Per Serving ■ Calories: 140 ■ Calories from fat: 61 (13% of tot cal) ■ % Daily Value* ■ Total Fat 7g 11% ■ Saturated Fat 3g 15% ■ Cholesterol 12mg 4% ■ Sodium 557mg 23% ■ Total Carbo 18g 6% ■ Dietary Fiber 5g 20% ■ Sugars 10g ■ Protein 2g ■ Vitamin A 1642% ■ Vitamin C 67% ■ Calcium 7% ■ Iron 9%

*Percent Daily Values are based on a 2000 calorie diet. Your daily values may be higher or lower depending upon your caloric intake.

Chicken Enchilada Casserole R

8 SERVINGS

As with Italian foods, Mexican foods are especially appealing to children (which might have something to do with the cheese!). This Mexican-inspired dish is easy and fun to make. When you have time, invite your children to help you assemble the casserole. If you've got more than one child, put each one in charge of one ingredient for layering. You can make the Santa Fe–Style Green Chile Sauce (page 184) a day or two ahead and refrigerate it until you're ready to assemble the casserole.

> 3 cups Santa Fe–Style Green Chile Sauce
> One 4-pound chicken
> 16 6-inch corn tortillas
> 4 to 5 cups (1 to 1¼ pounds) shredded Monterey Jack cheese

1. Make the Green Chile Sauce.
2. Place the chicken in a large pot, cover with cold water, and bring to a boil. Reduce to a simmer and skim the scum from the top of the water. Cook for 30 to 45 minutes or until cooked through. Allow the chicken to cool slightly before removing the meat from the bones. Discard the skin and bones and tear the meat into small pieces.
3. Preheat the oven to 350°F.
4. Assemble the casserole: spread a thin layer of sauce in the bottom of a 9 × 13-inch baking dish.
5. Add a layer of 8 tortillas. Cover completely with sauce. Add a layer of half the chicken, another layer of sauce, and a layer of half the cheese.
6. Repeat the layers, ending with cheese.
7. Bake for 20 to 30 minutes, until the casserole is heated through.

Santa Fe–Style Green Chile Sauce R

■

4 CUPS

The smell of roasting chiles permeates the air in Santa Fe during harvest season. As far back as the 1500s, Spanish explorers found chiles being cultivated in the area that is now New Mexico. Today, more land is dedicated to the cultivation of chiles in New Mexico than any other state. In fact, chiles are so important to New Mexicans that many families even grow their own and save seeds from year to year. This recipe brings the fragrance of roasted chiles to the plate and adds a little zip to your enchiladas.

½ cup Spanish onion (1 small), diced small

1 teaspoon minced garlic (1 clove)

1 tablespoon canola oil

2 tablespoons all-purpose flour

2 cups roasted, peeled, and chopped New Mexican green or poblano chiles

2 cups water

1 teaspoon kosher salt

¼ teaspoon freshly ground black pepper

1. In a large saucepan, sauté the onion and garlic in the oil.
2. Stir in the flour and continue cooking over moderate heat, stirring occasionally, for 15 to 20 minutes.
3. Add the chiles and water and cook over low heat until the sauce has turned to a deep green color and has no floury taste, about 20 to 30 minutes. Do not hurry this sauce—the flavors will develop more fully if the sauce is cooked slowly. Add the salt and pepper.

NUTRITION FACTS

Serving Size: ⅓ cup ■ Servings Per Recipe: 12 ■ Amount Per Serving ■ Calories: 28 ■ Calories from fat: 11 (39% of tot cal) ■ % Daily Value* ■ Total Fat 1g 2% ■ Saturated Fat 0g 0% ■ Cholesterol 0mg 0% ■ Sodium 200mg 8% ■ Total Carbo 4g 1% ■ Dietary Fiber 1g 2% ■ Sugars 2g ■ Protein 1g ■ Vitamin A 19% ■ Vitamin C 136% ■ Calcium 1% ■ Iron 4%

*Percent Daily Values are based on a 2000 calorie diet. Your daily values may be higher or lower depending upon your caloric intake.

Turkey Meatloaf R

8 SERVINGS

Meatloaf is an American comfort food. Some fondly remember their mother or grandmother making it for Sunday dinner and others remember it—uh—just a little less fondly. This recipe is made with ground turkey instead of ground beef, which lowers the saturated fat content of the meal, and if you follow this recipe you won't end up with a dried-out piece of shoe leather. It's surprisingly easy to prepare, too!

"This meatloaf was so delicious we ate it three days in a row.
I even made meatloaf sandwiches and it was just like eating
leftover Thanksgiving dinner!"

— NICOLE FINDLAY, HOUSTON, TX, MOTHER OF TWIN GIRLS

½ cup onion (1 small), diced small

¼ cup shredded carrot (1 medium)

1 teaspoon minced garlic (1 clove)

1 tablespoon canola oil

3 pounds ground turkey

1 teaspoon chopped parsley

½ cup Japanese bread crumbs (panko)

3 eggs

1 teaspoon kosher salt

¼ teaspoon freshly ground black pepper

3 tablespoons ketchup

1. Preheat the oven to 350°F. Prepare an 8 × 4-inch loaf pan.
2. In a small skillet, sauté onion, garlic, and carrot in the oil until soft. Remove from the heat and allow to cool slightly before transferring to a separate bowl.
3. Combine the sautéed ingredients with the turkey, parsley, bread crumbs, eggs, salt, and pepper and mix well.
4. Pack the mixture into the loaf pan, coat top with the ketchup, and bake to an internal temperature of 140°F (measure with an instant-read thermometer), about 45 to 60 minutes.

NUTRITION FACTS
Serving Size: 1-inch slice ▪ Servings Per Recipe: 8 ▪ Amount Per Serving ▪ Calories: 169 ▪ Calories from fat: 82 (49% of tot cal) ▪ % Daily Value* ▪ Total Fat 9g 14% ▪ Saturated Fat 2g 12% ▪ Cholesterol 113mg 38% ▪ Sodium 366mg 15% ▪ Total Carbo 4g 1% ▪ Dietary Fiber 0g 1% ▪ Sugars 1g ▪ Protein 17g ▪ Vitamin A 66% ▪ Vitamin C 2% ▪ Calcium 3% ▪ Iron 14%

*Percent Daily Values are based on a 2000 calorie diet. Your daily values may be higher or lower depending upon your caloric intake.

 A Chicken McNugget is mushed-up little bits of dozens of chickens, plus over 50 chemicals and additives.

Red Lentil Burgers R

8 SERVINGS

Vegetarian and vegan items were often on the menu of the Ross School. This recipe was always a favorite. These lentil patties are delicious as well as healthful, and can be served as a burger on a whole-grain bun, or as an entrée with rice and some grilled veggies.

1 pound (1½ cups) red lentils

5 cups salted water

1 cup minced onion (1 medium)

½ cup minced carrot (1 large)

2 teaspoons minced garlic (2 cloves)

Olive oil for the skillet

2 cups chopped crimini mushrooms

1 tablespoon chopped fresh oregano

½ teaspoon salt

⅛ teaspoon freshly ground black pepper

¾ cup Japanese bread crumbs (panko)

4½ teaspoons lemon juice

10 ounces tofu, pureed in a blender

1. In a large pot, boil the lentils in salted water until tender. Drain and cool.
2. In a large skillet, sauté the onion, carrot, and garlic in 1 teaspoon olive oil until tender, about 2 minutes.
3. Add the mushrooms, oregano, and salt and pepper to taste. Cook until mushrooms are tender and liquid has evaporated, approximately 5 minutes, and allow to cool.
4. Add the bread crumbs, lemon juice, pureed tofu, 2 tablespoons olive

oil and mix to combine. Transfer to a large bowl. Chill for 30 minutes and then shape into 8 patties.

5. Pan-fry in olive oil in a large skillet until each side is crisp and golden. Finish in a 350°F oven if necessary to heat through.

NUTRITION FACTS

Serving Size: 1 burger ■ Servings Per Recipe: 8 ■ Amount Per Serving ■ Calories: 151 ■ Calories from fat: 20 (13% of tot cal) ■ % Daily Value* ■ Total Fat 2g 3% ■ Saturated Fat 0g 1% ■ Cholesterol 0mg 0% ■ Sodium 164mg 7% ■ Total Carbo 33g 11% ■ Dietary Fiber 10g 38% ■ Sugars 3g ■ Protein 11g ■ Vitamin A 160% ■ Vitamin C 9% ■ Calcium 4% Iron 33%

*Percent Daily Values are based on a 2000 calorie diet. Your daily values may be higher or lower depending upon your caloric intake.

Lunchables™ Bite

They're a fun concept, and they're really easy for parents to buy and pack into a backpack for their kids' lunches, but they're composed of heavily processed foods. Earlier versions were absolutely loaded with fat, saturated fat, and cholesterol. These days, Oscar Mayer is sticking closer to the USDA's nutritional guidelines, but we still think parents would do better to steer clear of Lunchables in the grocery store because processed foods aren't good for your kids. Instead, assemble your own build-your-own-lunch. Using the Laptop Lunches system (see page 160) or something similar that you've put together yourself, you can pack similarly interactive lunches for your kids, using wholesome, healthful, organic ingredients. Try mini-taco lunches using baked tortilla chips, seasoned chicken, shredded cheese, and guacamole. Cut whole-wheat pita bread into triangles or circles using a 2-inch circle cutter (star shapes are great for little kids, too) and put those in a lunch box with home-cooked meats, cheese, a condiment or two, or just plain nut butter and 100 percent fruit jelly. Pack bread, along with carrot, red bell pepper, and celery sticks and Ranch dressing or even our Broccoli Pesto (see page 212) or include the ingredients for a salad and let your child put it together at school. Sure, Lunchables are faster, but they're expensive and you can't customize them. When you make your own you can choose foods you know your child will love and, just to keep him on his toes, you can throw in something new!

Mac and Cheese CPF

8 SERVINGS

"This was the all-time best recipe ever. Seriously. It's not only
the best mac and cheese recipe; it's not only the best recipe
I've tested; it's the best food of all time. Everyone loved it."

— LISA MACON, ORLANDO, FL

You'll be surprised by how easy this macaroni is to prepare, so even if
you have very little cooking experience you'll have no trouble with this
recipe. For kids who don't like "crusty" macaroni and cheese, this need
not go in the oven—just follow the recipe through step 6 and serve. It's
also easier to send this to school in a thermos without the crusty top.

1 pound elbow macaroni
8 tablespoons (1 stick) unsalted butter
½ cup all-purpose flour, sifted
3 cups 1% milk
1 cup (4 ounces) shredded Cheddar cheese
1 cup (4 ounces) shredded Monterey Jack cheese

1. If you'll be making it crusty, preheat the oven to 350°F. In a large
   stockpot, bring salted water to a boil for cooking the pasta.
2. While waiting for the pasta water to boil, melt the butter in a large
   saucepan. Add the flour and cook, stirring occasionally, for 10
   minutes.
3. Stir in the milk gradually and bring to boil. Reduce to simmer and
   cook for 15 minutes.
4. While the sauce is simmering, boil the macaroni in the salted water
   until al dente, according to package directions.

5. While the pasta is cooking, stir the cheeses into the sauce until fully melted and remove from the heat.

6. When the pasta has finished cooking, drain it in a colander and add it to the cheese sauce. Mix to combine.

7. Pour it into a 9 × 13-inch baking dish and bake for 30 minutes. Allow to cool slightly and serve hot.

NUTRITION FACTS

Serving Size: 1 cup ▪ Servings Per Recipe: 8 ▪ Amount Per Serving ▪ Calories: 490 ▪ Calories from fat: 219 (45% of tot cal) ▪ % Daily Value* ▪ Total Fat 24g 38% ▪ Saturated Fat 15g 75% ▪ Cholesterol 71mg 24% ▪ Sodium 1804mg 75% ▪ Total Carbo 50g 17% ▪ Dietary Fiber 2g 6% ▪ Sugars 5g ▪ Protein 18g ▪ Vitamin A 83% ▪ Vitamin C 2% ▪ Calcium 36% Iron 6%

*Percent Daily Values are based on a 2000 calorie diet. Your daily values may be higher or lower depending upon your caloric intake.

Squash Phyllo Triangles CPF

4 SERVINGS

Phyllo (literally translated, "leaf") dough, popular in Greek and Middle Eastern cuisine, is often avoided by the average home cook because it seems so delicate and difficult to use. In reality, even though it is quite fragile, it is also very forgiving. Most often layered and brushed with butter or olive oil, the dough doesn't show rips and tears the way a pie crust might. The best thing about phyllo dough is that it will make you look like a culinary genius because it's so light and flaky. Phyllo dough is so thin it will dry out quickly if left at room temperature, so cover unused dough with a damp cloth as you work.

These can be served at room temperature and are an interesting and very portable packed lunch item. They freeze well—make several batches and put them in plastic freezer bags.

2 tablespoons olive oil

3 cloves garlic, minced

1 medium yellow squash, grated

1 medium zucchini, grated

½ cup lightly packed basil leaves, washed and chopped

⅓ cup crumbled feta cheese

1 large egg, beaten

4 tablespoons (½ stick) unsalted butter, melted

2 sheets phyllo dough

1. Preheat the oven to 350°F.
2. Heat the oil in a large skillet. Add the garlic, squashes, and basil and sauté for 5 to 8 minutes or until tender.
3. Remove from the heat and transfer squash mixture to a medium bowl to cool.
4. Add the feta cheese and egg and mix well.
5. Place a sheet of phyllo dough on a dry surface and brush lightly with butter. Top with the second sheet and brush with butter.
6. Cut the sheet lengthwise into quarters and place one-quarter of the filling at one end of each strip.
7. Fold each strip as you would a flag and brush the tops with butter. Bake on a cookie sheet for 10 to 15 minutes or until golden.

NUTRITION FACTS

Serving Size: 1 triangle ■ Servings Per Recipe: 4 ■ Amount Per Serving ■ Calories: 183 ■ Calories from fat: 117 (64% of tot cal) ■ % Daily Value* ■ Total Fat 13g 20% ■ Saturated Fat 4g 22% ■ Cholesterol 78mg 26% ■ Sodium 278mg 12% ■ Total Carbo 11g 4% ■ Dietary Fiber 2g 7% ■ Sugars 3g ■ Protein 7g ■ Vitamin A 63% ■ Vitamin C 29% ■ Calcium 15% ■ Iron 13%

*Percent Daily Values are based on a 2,000 calorie diet. Your daily values may be higher or lower depending upon your caloric intake.

 McDonald's french fries have little in common with a potato: They contain more than 10 ingredients, including flavoring that comes from a beef source and, of course, trans fats, sugar, and salt.

CSA: Community Supported Agriculture

A farm literally supported by its community, a CSA is an increasingly popular way for small farmers to stay in business without giving in to more conventional and destructive farming methods. In 1990, there were only about fifty known CSAs in the United States. Today that number has grown to over 1,000. Participants are ordinarily asked to choose among a variety of membership options. A person, or family, is required to purchase a "share" before the season begins, which entitles the purchaser to weekly or biweekly pickups (in some cases, deliveries) of fresh—often organic—produce.

The average cost per share varies according to region and the consumer's level of participation on the farm during the season, but most family shares can be purchased for an average of between $350 and $600. A person willing to work on the farm a few hours a week can purchase a part-time work share at a reduced rate. A full-time work share requires the purchasers to work many more hours but entitles them to an entire season of free produce (in most cases). No matter which option a person chooses, it's an incredible deal.

Research has determined that the average CSA share yields approximately 400 pounds of produce for the season. Consumers buying an equivalent amount of organic produce in a store could expect to pay upwards of $1,000. The same amount of conventionally raised produce would cost between $680 and $780, translating to savings of $200 to $450 for CSA members. Setting the system up this way is clearly beneficial to the consumer who has a new opportunity to become part of an agricultural community through hands-on farming experience. Most CSAs will allow older children to participate in a family work share, and some even offer special classes for kids. There's no better way for your child to learn about where his food comes from, and it helps the farmers who are the most important link in our food chain. Buying shares in advance gives farmers the necessary capital to purchase seeds and supplies. It also saves biologically diverse farms that might ultimately disappear due to an inability to compete with large monocropping farms and the temptation to sell out to agribusiness.

CSA participation is not limited to rural areas. In New York City, consumers looking for organic food products can employ the services of Urban Organics, a distributor of organic produce, groceries, and dairy goods. Organized more along the lines of an organic food club, Urban Organics asks its customers to purchase a membership, which allows them to choose from a menu of items. Boxes of fruits and vegetables are provided in various sizes to suit the needs of a particular household. Like typical rural CSAs, what arrives at the consumer's door is dependent upon the seasons. Unfortunately, however, members do not have the option to work on a farm.

Snapshot of a CSA

Scott Chaskey runs Quail Hill Farm on Long Island in New York. CSA members adore Scott. He gives great hugs, has the most wonderful eyes, a fantastic beard, grows incredible food, and is utterly passionate about what he does. And what he does is grow organic food on land owned by the Peconic Land Trust, a nonprofit group working to conserve land on Long Island. Since it was established in 1990, Quail Hill Farm has grown to twenty-five acres serving 150 local families. Farm members purchase a share each year, which enables them to harvest fresh vegetables, fruits, and flowers throughout the growing season. In addition to Scott, the preserve manager, the Trust employs four apprentices to plant the crops, care for the fields, and assist farm members.

One year Ann had the good fortune of being a member of Quail Hill Farm and experienced it as a wonderful, soulful, enriching, and delicious experience. Once or twice a week she would drive or ride her bike over to the farm and pick her share of the food for that week. The experience of understanding the time and place of our food—that tomatoes don't really ripen until August, that strawberries are only available in June, and that raspberries are a treat literally all summer long—is the most valuable lesson people take with them from a CSA. Every week, families, single adults, children, and people of all ages would be walking the rows with their bags and baskets picking the fresh vegetables, soaking in the sun (or the rain), gathering recipes from the farm stand, and enjoying this unique way to participate in producing and harvesting their own food. Nothing brings a community together the way food does, and a CSA is one of the best ways to teach your children about food and farming.

Chile Cornbread R

9 SERVINGS

This cornbread recipe can be a snack, a side to Vegetarian Black Bean Chili (page 180), or even part of a balanced breakfast. It is a great complement to egg dishes, including spicy Southwestern breakfast burritos. Sweet pepper jam or jelly make healthier alternatives to butter.

5 tablespoons unsalted butter

½ cup yellow cornmeal

¼ cup all-purpose flour

⅓ cup cake flour

1 tablespoon + 1½ teaspoons white corn flour

2 tablespoons sugar

1 teaspoon baking powder

½ teaspoon kosher salt

2 tablespoons + ¾ teaspoon 1% milk

6 tablespoons buttermilk

1 cup large egg, beaten

¼ cup fresh corn kernels (1 ear)

2 tablespoons + 1½ teaspoons roasted and roughly chopped green chile pepper

1. Preheat oven to 350°F. Grease an 8 × 8-inch baking pan with butter.
2. Melt the butter and cool.
3. Combine the cornmeal, flours, sugar, baking powder, and salt in a medium bowl and set aside.
4. In another bowl, combine milk, buttermilk, butter, and egg and blend thoroughly. Add the liquid ingredients to the dry ingredients and mix well. Stir in the corn and chiles.

5. Pour the batter into the prepared pan and bake for 20 to 30 minutes, or until a toothpick comes out clean. Cut into squares and serve. The cornbread can be stored at room temperature in an airtight container for up to 3 days.

NUTRITION FACTS

Serving Size: One 2½ × 2½-inch piece ■ Servings Per Recipe: 9 ■ Amount Per Serving ■ Calories: 150 ■ Calories from fat: 68 (45% of tot cal) ■ % Daily Value* ■ Total Fat 8g 12% ■ Saturated Fat 4g 22% ■ Cholesterol 45mg 15% ■ Sodium 60mg 2% ■ Total Carbo 18g 6% ■ Dietary Fiber 1g 4% ■ Sugars 4g ■ Protein 3g ■ Vitamin A 34% ■ Vitamin C 9% ■ Calcium 7% ■ Iron 12%

*Percent Daily Values are based on a 2000 calorie diet. Your daily values may be higher or lower depending upon your caloric intake.

Arugula with Steak, Lemon, and Parmesan R

8 SERVINGS

This is one of our favorite salads. We love the flavor combination of the spicy arugula, the clean citrus, and the grilled flavor of the meat—not to mention the Parmesan! It's important to buy hormone- and antibiotic-free meat, and since there are so few ingredients, make sure that your olive oil and balsamic vinegar are of especially good quality so the flavors will be well-developed. This is probably best served at home for lunch, but it can also be sent in a lunch box as long as the greens aren't dressed ahead of time—send the dressing on the side.

 There are more than 400 school districts with farm-to-cafeteria programs in 22 states nationwide.

3 tablespoons extra virgin olive oil

2½ teaspoons lemon juice

1¼ teaspoons balsamic vinegar

Dash kosher salt

Dash freshly ground black pepper

1½ pounds beef tri-tip (bottom sirloin)

1 bunch (about 5½ cups) arugula

¾ cup Parmesan cheese, shaved

1. To make the dressing, combine the olive oil, lemon juice, balsamic vinegar, salt, and pepper. Set aside.
2. Grill the beef to medium rare, let cool 10 minutes. Slice thin.
3. Toss the arugula with the dressing and add beef and shaved Parmesan.

NUTRITION FACTS

Serving Size: 3 oz meat and ¾ cup salad ■ Servings Per Recipe: 8 ■ Amount Per Serving ■ Calories: 236 ■ Calories from fat: 163 (69% of tot cal) ■ % Daily Value* ■ Total Fat 18g 28% ■ Saturated Fat 7g 36% ■ Cholesterol 43mg 14% ■ Sodium 373mg 16% ■ Total Carbo 2g 1% ■ Dietary Fiber 0g 2% ■ Sugars 1g ■ Protein 16g ■ Vitamin A 80% ■ Vitamin C 11% ■ Calcium 33% ■ Iron 14%

*Percent Daily Values are based on a 2000 calorie diet. Your daily values may be higher or lower depending upon your caloric intake.

Salade Niçoise R

8 SERVINGS

Salade niçoise is a classic. Fresh, clean flavors of boiled potatoes, green beans, hard-boiled eggs, and recently caught fish make it a spring favorite for lunch or dinner. Line-caught tuna is the preferred environmentally friendly choice, but this salad can also be made with canned tuna. Be sure to buy dolphin-free, water-packed light meat only, for the best flavor and the most environmentally safe choice. (See page 22 for more about mercury in fish). Salade niçoise is delicious at room temperature and benefits from a little marination, so it makes a terrific lunch box meal. Note that the fish is cooked a day ahead, so plan accordingly.

1 pound fresh tuna

1 cup canola oil

2 sprigs fresh thyme

1 clove garlic, peeled

¼ teaspoon whole fennel seeds, toasted

¼ teaspoon black peppercorns, toasted

Kosher salt

1 cup extra virgin olive oil

1 tablespoon Dijon mustard

½ cup red wine vinegar

2 tablespoons minced shallots (1 medium)

Freshly ground black pepper

4 large eggs

½ pound green beans

1 pound baby red potatoes

2 large fresh tomatoes, cut in wedges

¼ pound niçoise olives, pitted

2 tablespoons capers, drained and rinsed

2-ounce can anchovy filets, drained and patted dry

1 pound Boston lettuce (2 heads)

1. *The day before:* Place the tuna in heavy-bottomed pan with the canola oil, thyme, garlic, fennel seed, and peppercorns, and some salt. Heat to 160 degrees (check with an instant-read thermometer) and cook the fish until it is no longer pink. Remove the tuna from the pan, place in a clean container, strain the oil over the tuna and let cool in refrigerator about 1 hour. Discard the flavorings.

2. *The next day:* Prepare the vinaigrette by whisking together the extra virgin olive oil, Dijon mustard, and red wine vinegar. Once the mixture is emulsified (meaning the oil and vinegar have come together and the mixture has thickened) add the shallots and season with salt and pepper.

3. Hard boil the eggs and steam the green beans and potatoes. Cut the potatoes into chunks, break the tuna into bite-size pieces, and peel and halve the eggs. Pour vinaigrette over tuna, beans, potatoes, eggs, and tomatoes. Top with the capers, olives, and anchovies.

4. For serving at home, place the lettuce on a plate and top with salad. To send to school, place lettuce in a plastic container with prepared salad niçoise on top and then turn it upside down so that the lettuce doesn't get soggy.

NUTRITION FACTS

Serving Size: 1 oz tuna and 7.5 oz vegetables ■ Servings Per Recipe: 8 ■ Amount Per Serving ■ Calories: 324 ■ Calories from fat: 176 (54% of tot cal) ■ % Daily Value* ■ Total Fat 20g 30% ■ Saturated Fat 3g 16% ■ Cholesterol 142mg 47% ■ Sodium 597mg 25% ■ Total Carbo 22g 7% ■ Dietary Fiber 5g 21% ■ Sugars 2g ■ Protein 17g ■ Vitamin A 93% ■ Vitamin C 66% ■ Calcium 10% ■ Iron 28%

*Percent Daily Values are based on a 2,000 calorie diet. Your daily values may be higher or lower depending upon your caloric intake.

Baked Pasta with Tomato and Ricotta R

8 SERVINGS

This is a recipe that kids seem to love. It can be set up the night before or in the morning and baked just prior to mealtime. Leftovers even taste good cold! We often add sautéed vegetables to this dish. In the spring try mushrooms and fresh greens. Later in the season, zucchini and summer squash make tasty additions.

"The pasta was excellent! The kids were sooooo tired after having a sleepover with their cousins and then starting school and they were very cranky before dinner. Maddie asked what was for dinner and when I told her they all started crying that they don't even like that. They then proceeded to DEVOUR more than half the pan!! They LOVED it. This recipe will be added to our favorites for sure."

—MICHELLE WIESNER, AURORA, CO, MOTHER OF FOUR

1 pound any variety of dry pasta

1 tablespoon shredded mozzarella cheese

½ cup ricotta cheese

2 tablespoons grated Parmesan cheese

1 large egg, beaten (you may need another)

1 teaspoon kosher salt

½ teaspoon freshly ground black pepper

2½ cups Basic Tomato Sauce (page 200)

1. Cook pasta very al dente.
2. Preheat oven to 350°F.
3. In a small bowl, beat together the ricotta, 1 tablespoon of Parmesan, the beaten egg, salt, and pepper. The mixture should be loose and easy to scoop. If it is too firm, add an additional egg.
3. In a 9 × 13-inch baking dish, layer sauce, pasta, and ricotta. Repeat the layers. Top casserole with the grated mozzarella and the remaining Parmesan. Bake for 20 minutes or until the cheese is melted and bubbly.

NUTRITION FACTS

Serving Size: 1 cup ■ Servings Per Recipe: 8 ■ Amount Per Serving ■ Calories: 151 ■ Calories from fat: 46 (30% of tot cal) ■ % Daily Value* ■ Total fat 5g 8% ■ Saturated Fat 2g 10% ■ Cholesterol 62mg 21% ■ Sodium 709mg 30% ■ Total Carbo 18g 6% ■ Dietary Fiber 1g 4% ■ Sugars 0g ■ Protein 8g ■ Vitamin A 40% ■ Vitamin C 13% ■ Calcium 12% ■ Iron 17%

*Percent Daily Values are based on a 2000 calorie diet. Your daily values may be higher or lower depending upon your caloric intake.

Basic Tomato Sauce R

8 SERVINGS

Tomato sauce is ubiquitous in American cuisine. Whether served with pasta, as an ingredient in lasagna, or as a side with grilled chicken, tomato sauce is a part of many types of meals. This tomato sauce is the perfect ingredient for any of the above-mentioned dishes. If you're feeling particularly industrious, make a double batch and freeze half for later use.

4½ teaspoons Spanish onion, diced small
1 clove garlic, minced
1 teaspoon extra virgin olive oil
3½ cups (28-ounce can) canned diced tomatoes
½ bay leaf
1½ teaspoons chopped fresh oregano
1½ teaspoons thinly sliced fresh basil

1. In a medium nonreactive saucepan over medium-low heat, sauté the onion and garlic in olive oil until translucent.
2. Add the tomatoes and bay leaf and simmer until the flavors are blended about 1 hour.
3. Stir in the oregano and basil. Remove the bay leaf. This sauce may be served as is or pureed, whichever you prefer.

NUTRITION FACTS

Serving Size: ½ cup ▪ Servings Per Recipe: 8 ▪ Amount Per Serving ▪ Calories: 37 ▪ Calories from fat: 14 (38% of tot cal) ▪ % Daily Value* ▪ Total Fat 2g 2% ▪ Saturated Fat 0g 2% ▪ Cholesterol 0mg 0% ▪ Sodium 174mg 7% ▪ Total Carbo 5g 2% ▪ Dietary Fiber 1g 4% ▪ Sugars 0g ▪ Protein 1g ▪ Vitamin A 33% ▪ Vitamin C 19% ▪ Calcium 2% ▪ Iron 6%

*Percent Daily Values are based on a 2000 calorie diet. Your daily values may be higher or lower depending upon your caloric intake.

Spinach Salad with Tangerines R

■

4 SERVINGS

Sweet and tangy, this salad can be eaten on its own or with the addition of grilled or roasted seafood, chicken, pork, or beef. Oranges and grapefruit can be substituted for the tangerines, and arugula, watercress, or mâche make a flavorful addition to the spinach. If you're packing it for lunch, put the dressing in a small plastic container so the salad won't wilt.

1 cup red onion (1 medium), sliced thin

1 teaspoon rice vinegar

1½ cups fresh spinach, leaves only, tightly packed

1½ cups frisée lettuce, tightly packed

1 cup tangerine sections

¼ cup Sesame-Ginger Vinaigrette (page 202)

Salt and freshly ground black pepper to taste

½ teaspoon toasted sesame seeds

1. In a large bowl, combine the onion and rice vinegar.
2. Add the greens and tangerines and toss with Sesame Ginger Vinaigrette. Adjust seasoning. Garnish with sesame seeds.

NUTRITION FACTS

Serving Size: 1 tablespoon dressing and 1 cup salad ■ Servings Per Recipe: 4 ■ Amount Per Serving ■ Calories: 136 ■ Calories from fat: 92 (68% of tot cal) ■ % Daily Value* ■ Total Fat 10g 16% ■ Saturated Fat 1g 5% ■ Cholesterol 0mg 0% ■ Sodium 157mg 7% ■ Total Carbo 12g 4% ■ Dietary Fiber 3g 10% ■ Sugars 8g ■ Protein 1g ■ Vitamin A 131% ■ Vitamin C 50% ■ Calcium 4% ■ Iron 6%

*Percent Daily Values are based on a 2000 calorie diet. Your daily values may be higher or lower depending upon your caloric intake.

 The direct and indirect medical costs of obesity now consume more than 10 percent of the U.S. health care budget.

Sesame-Ginger Vinaigrette R

2 CUPS

This dressing is perfect for Spinach Salad with Tangerines (page 201), but it would also work well on an Asian-inspired pasta salad or in a chicken or pork sandwich wrap with tender greens.

3 tablespoons chopped fresh ginger

¾ cup rice vinegar

3 tablespoons soy sauce

¾ cup canola oil

3 tablespoons sesame oil

2 teaspoons grated orange zest

1. Combine all the ingredients, except the zest, in a blender and blend to emulsify.
2. Stir in the orange zest.

NUTRITION FACTS
Serving Size: 1 tablespoon ■ Servings Per Recipe: 32 ■ Amount Per Serving ■ Calories: 59 ■ Calories from fat: 58 (98% of tot cal) ■ % Daily Value* ■ Total Fat 6g 10% ■ Saturated Fat 1g 3% ■ Cholesterol 0mg 0% ■ Sodium 94mg 4% ■ Total Carbo 1g 0% ■ Dietary Fiber 0g 0% ■ Sugars 0g ■ Protein 0g ■ Vitamin A 0% ■ Vitamin C 0% ■ Calcium 0% Iron 1%

*Percent Daily Values are based on a 2000 calorie diet. Your daily values may be higher or lower depending upon your caloric intake.

Kaiser Permanente, the largest health care organization in the United States, recently started hosting farmers' markets and sourcing local healthy foods at many of its properties.

Spring Soup CPF

8 SERVINGS

From a culinary standpoint, spring can be the hardest time of year. Tired of the dense, starchy root vegetables of winter, cooks are ready for early greens, pea shoots, asparagus—and fresh, light flavors. Yet what's actually available is often a bit less inspiring. This recipe helps bring spring to the table even when a chill is still in the air.

1 pound small new potatoes, cut in medium pieces

2 cups water

2½ teaspoons kosher salt

¼ teaspoon freshly ground black pepper

2 tablespoons unsalted butter

4 small scallions (green onions), thinly sliced

½ pound baby carrots, small diced

2 cups half-and-half

3 tablespoons all-purpose flour

3 cups shelled peas (about 3 pounds in the pod)

1. Cook the potatoes in simmering water for 5 minutes. They will not be tender. Add the salt, pepper, butter, scallions, and carrots and simmer 5 minutes more.
2. In a small mixing bowl, combine the half-and-half and flour and stir until smooth. Add to soup pot, mixing well. Cook 5 minutes.
3. Add the peas, cook for 2 minutes more, and serve.

NUTRITION FACTS

Serving Size: About 1 cup ■ Servings Per Recipe: 8 ■ Amount Per Serving ■ Calories: 201 ■ Calories from fat: 91 (45% of tot cal) ■ % Daily Value* ■ Total Fat 10g 16% ■ Saturated Fat 6g 31% ■ Cholesterol

30mg 10% ■ Sodium 810mg 34% ■ Total Carbo 23g 8% ■ Dietary Fiber 4g 17% ■ Sugars 2g ■
Protein 5g ■ Vitamin A 893% ■ Vitamin C 64% ■ Calcium 13% ■ Iron 21%

*Percent Daily Values are based on a 2000 calorie diet. Your daily values may be higher or lower depending upon your caloric intake.

Chicken Caesar Wrap R

6 SERVINGS

Wraps have become some of the great "to-go" foods of our times—they seem suddenly to be everywhere. If packing this wrap in the morning for lunch at school, either dress it lightly or consider serving the dressing on the side. If you send the dressing on the side you can make the wrap the night before, which will free you up to make a more complicated breakfast meal (or just relax with your cup of coffee!) in the morning.

1½ cups shredded romaine lettuce
6 tablespoons Caesar Dressing (page 205)
Salt and freshly ground black pepper
1½ pounds roast chicken (meat only), shredded
6 6-inch flour tortillas

1. Toss the lettuce in a medium bowl with the Caesar dressing. Taste and adjust seasoning with salt and pepper if necessary.
2. Place 4 ounces of chicken at the center of each tortilla and top each with ¼ cup of salad. Fold ends in, roll, and serve.

NUTRITION FACTS

Serving Size: 1 wrap ■ Servings Per Recipe: 6 ■ Amount Per Serving ■ Calories: 320 ■ Calories from fat: 116 (43% of tot cal) ■ % Daily Value* ■ Total Fat 13g 20% ■ Saturated Fat 2g 10% ■ Cholesterol 74mg 25% ■ Sodium 481mg 20% ■ Total Carbo 27g 9% ■ Dietary Fiber 0g 1% ■ Sugars 0g ■ Protein 23g ■ Vitamin A 51% ■ Vitamin C 13% ■ Calcium 13% ■ Iron 28%

Caesar Dressing R

2 CUPS

Any dressing can be packed in a school lunch to be used as a dip for vegetables. This traditional Caesar dressing is sure to become a family favorite no matter how you serve it.

2 pasteurized egg yolks
1 tablespoon red wine vinegar
1 tablespoon lemon juice
1 clove garlic, chopped
2 tablespoons Dijon mustard
¼ cup Worcestershire sauce
¼ cup chopped anchovies
1 cup olive oil
¼ teaspoon kosher salt
⅛ teaspoon ground black pepper

In a food processor, blend all ingredients except the oil, salt, and pepper. When the mixture is smooth, drizzle the oil in a thin stream while the processor is running to emulsify the dressing. Adjust the seasoning with salt and pepper if necessary.

NUTRITION FACTS

Serving Size: 1 tablespoon ■ Servings Per Recipe: 32 ■ Amount Per Serving ■ Calories: 70 ■ Calories from fat: 65 (93% of tot cal) ■ % Daily Value* ■ Total Fat 7g 11% ■ Saturated Fat 1g 5% ■ Cholesterol 15mg 5% ■ Sodium 117mg 5% ■ Total Carbo 1g 0% ■ Dietary Fiber 0g 0% ■ Sugars 0g ■ Protein 1g ■ Vitamin A 2% ■ Vitamin C 1% ■ Calcium 1% ■ Iron 2%

*Percent Daily Values are based on a 2000 calorie diet. Your daily values may be higher or lower depending upon your caloric intake.

Couscous with Tofu, Zucchini, and Basil R

4 SERVINGS

Couscous is a delicious and delicate grain that should be in every parent's pantry because it's so versatile and easy to make. This recipe can be served warm or cold, as an entrée with the addition of grilled chicken, fish, or pork, or as a side dish. Experiment with couscous—try substituting savory ingredients with sweet ones, like raisins, dried cranberries or apricots, and nuts.

2 cups water, salted

1/3 cup couscous

6 tablespoons olive oil

2¾ ounces (½ cup) firm tofu, diced small

2 tablespoons lemon juice

½ clove garlic, sliced thin (1 medium)

½ cup seeded zucchini, diced small

½ cup red onion (½ small), diced small

¾ cup thinly sliced fresh basil

¼ cup chopped Italian flat-leaf parsley

1 teaspoon grated lemon zest

½ teaspoon ground red chili

 When buying their own food and drink, half of kids 7 to 12 choose candy, more than one-third choose soda and ice cream, and about one-quarter fast food.

1. Bring two cups of salted water to a boil.
2. Place raw couscous in a large bowl and add enough of the salted boiling water to just cover the couscous. Allow it to stand about 20 minutes or until the liquid is absorbed.
3. Drizzle 3 tablespoons of the olive oil into the couscous and use fork to break up lumps (you may need to use your hands).
4. In a small bowl, combine the remaining oil, tofu, lemon juice, and garlic, and pour over the tofu. Set aside.
5. Add the zucchini, onion, herbs, zest, and ground chili to the couscous and mix well. Drain the tofu and gently toss into the couscous. Adjust seasoning if necessary.

NUTRITION FACTS

Serving Size: About 3.25 ounces ■ Servings Per Recipe: 4 ■ Amount Per Serving ■ Calories: 83 ■ Calories from fat: 7 (8% of tot cal) ■ % Daily Value* ■ Total Fat 1g 1% ■ Saturated Fat 0g 1% ■ Cholesterol 0mg 0% ■ Sodium 12mg 1% ■ Total Carbo 16g 5% ■ Dietary Fiber 2g 7% ■ Sugars 2g ■ Protein 4g ■ Vitamin A 61% ■ Vitamin C 33% ■ Calcium 4% Iron 10%

*Percent Daily Values are based on a 2000 calorie diet. Your daily values may be higher or lower depending upon your caloric intake.

Oven Fried Chicken R

8 SERVINGS

Fried chicken is an American institution. It's everywhere, and let's face it, it's good. At the Ross School the chefs wanted to be able to serve fried chicken but needed to find a way to make a more healthful version. They did, and this is it, and it's better than some of the deep-fried versions. The best part? No oily mess in the kitchen afterward. Plan ahead, though: The chicken should be marinated overnight to allow the buttermilk enough time to tenderize the meat. Make it for dinner and send it to school cold the next day for lunch.

1½ cups buttermilk

2 teaspoons kosher salt

1 teaspoon freshly ground black pepper

3 pounds chicken cut into 8 pieces

1½ cups dry bread crumbs

¾ cup all-purpose flour

¾ cup cornmeal

¾ teaspoon chili powder

¼ teaspoon paprika

1. *The night before:* In a large bowl, mix the buttermilk, 1 teaspoon salt, and ½ teaspoon pepper. Marinate chicken in the buttermilk mixture overnight in the refrigerator.

2. *The next day:* Combine the bread crumbs, flour, cornmeal, chili powder, paprika, and remaining salt and pepper in a large bowl. Mix well.

3. Remove chicken from the marinade and roll in the bread-crumb mixture. If it's very wet, place it on a cooling rack set over a cookie sheet and allow to dry in the refrigerator for 1 to 3 hours (see Note).

4. Preheat the oven to 350°F.

5. Place the chicken directly on a cookie sheet and bake for 30 to 45 minutes or to an internal temperature of 145 degrees (check a few pieces with an instant-read thermometer).

Note: If you allow the bread crumb coating to dry in the refrigerator, be careful that it doesn't get overly dry, as it may burn in the oven. If it does dry out, just spray with water before putting it in the oven.

NUTRITION FACTS

Serving Size: 1 piece ■ Servings Per Recipe: 8 ■ Amount Per Serving ■ Calories: 382 ■ Calories from fat: 57 (15% of tot cal) ■ % Daily Value* ■ Total Fat 6g 10% ■ Saturated Fat 2g 8% ■ Cholesterol 120mg 40% ■ Sodium 1340mg 56% ■ Total Carbo 36g 12% ■ Dietary Fiber 2g 9% ■ Sugars 1g ■ Protein 42g ■ Vitamin A 24% ■ Vitamin C 10% ■ Calcium 7% ■ Iron 34%

*Percent Daily Values are based on a 2000 calorie diet. Your daily values may be higher or lower depending upon your caloric intake.

Red Bean Stew CPF

8 SERVINGS

Most people don't eat enough legumes. We're not talking about canned baked beans here—we're all about the bags of dried beans you pass on your way to pick up a box of rice. Over the years we've come to love beans. They're colorful, flavorful, and their nutritional benefits are unparalleled. High in fiber, legumes work to lower cholesterol, and paired with rice they make a virtually fat-free complete protein. When sending to school in a wide-mouthed vacuum bottle, either slightly undercook the rice and mix it in or cook the rice through and send it on the side.

2 cups dried kidney beans

3 cloves garlic

2 Spanish onions

5 carrots

¼ cup olive oil

1 bay leaf

4 sprigs fresh thyme

½ teaspoon red pepper flakes

½ teaspoon ground coriander seed

½ teaspoon cumin seed

2 cups Tomato Sauce (page 200)

2½ quarts vegetable stock

2 bunches Swiss chard, roughly chopped

Salt

 In 2000, government agencies spent about $48 million to promote nutrition and health for kids, but McDonald's spent 14 times that amount—$665 million—to advertise its food.

Freshly ground pepper

Cooked rice

1. Cook the kidney beans in water to cover until soft, approximately 2 to 4 hours at a simmer. (The beans may also be soaked overnight and will cook in about half the time.) Drain.
2. Peel and chop the garlic, onions, and carrots.
3. Heat the oil in a stockpot or large saucepan and sauté the garlic, onions, carrots, bay leaf, thyme, pepper flakes, coriander, and cumin for 5 minutes over medium heat.
4. Add the cooked kidney beans and tomato sauce.
5. Add the vegetable stock and chopped chard and simmer 8 to 10 minutes, until all flavors are well blended.
6. Add salt and pepper to taste and serve with rice.

NUTRITION FACTS

Serving Size: 1 cup ■ Servings Per Recipe: 8 ■ Amount Per Serving ■ Calories: 217 ■ Calories from fat: 70 (32% of tot cal) ■ % Daily Value* ■ Total Fat 8g 12% ■ Saturated Fat 1g 5% ■ Cholesterol 0mg 0% ■ Sodium 942mg 39% ■ Total Carbo 32g 11% ■ Dietary Fiber 9g 35% ■ Sugars 8g ■ Protein 8g ■ Vitamin A 3825% ■ Vitamin C 138% ■ Calcium 14% ■ Iron 41%

*Percent Daily Values are based on a 2000 calorie diet. Your daily values may be higher or lower depending upon your caloric intake.

Roasted Lemon-Herb Chicken R

8 SERVINGS

One of the biggest complaints about chicken is that the breast tends to dry out during cooking. In this recipe, brining the meat overnight makes it moist and extremely flavorful. If you decide to use boneless chicken it's only necessary to brine it for 2 to 3 hours. In the mood for something different? Try lemon thyme, lavender, or any other fresh herbs you have in the garden in place of the oregano, parsley, and basil in this recipe. This is a good choice for school lunch as long as your child's lunch box contains an ice pack.

1 tablespoon + 1½ teaspoons lemon juice

2 tablespoons kosher salt

2 quarts water

1½ pounds bone-in chicken parts (8 pieces)

1¾ teaspoons extra virgin olive oil

2 tablespoons chopped fresh oregano

2 tablespoons chopped Italian flat-leaf parsley

2 tablespoons thinly sliced fresh basil

⅛ teaspoon freshly ground black pepper

1. *The night before:* Combine the lemon juice, salt, and water in a large bowl. Add the chicken pieces, cover, and refrigerate overnight.

2. *The next day:* Remove the chicken from the brine and pat dry. In a clean large bowl, combine the oil, herbs, and pepper. Add the chicken and coat well. Cover and refrigerate for 4 to 6 hours to marinate.

3. Preheat the oven to 350°F.

4. Place the chicken pieces on a cookie sheet and bake for 30 to 45 minutes.

NUTRITION FACTS

Serving Size: 1 piece ■ Servings Per Recipe: 8 ■ Amount Per Serving ■ Calories: 124 ■ Calories from fat: 44 (35% of tot cal) ■ % Daily Value* ■ Total Fat 5g 7% ■ Saturated Fat 1g 5% ■ Cholesterol 59mg 20% ■ Sodium 1834mg 76% ■ Total Carbo 1g 0% ■ Dietary Fiber 1g 2% ■ Sugars 0g ■ Protein 18g ■ Vitamin A 20% ■ Vitamin C 12% ■ Calcium 4% ■ Iron 14%

*Percent Daily Values are based on a 2000 calorie diet. Your daily values may be higher or lower depending upon your caloric intake.

In 2004, the Associated Press reported that Krispy Kreme stores would give Palm Beach County (Florida) students in kindergarten through 6th grade a free doughnut for every A on their report card.

Broccoli Pesto CPF

■

8 SERVINGS

Most people associate pesto with basil, but it can be made with any number of green herbs, or even vegetables. This version, made with broccoli, is perfect on pasta, tastes great as a topping for grilled tofu, gets glowing reviews on grilled chicken or fish, and even works as a salad dressing. We like to use it on just about everything!

2 cups steamed and chopped broccoli
¼ cup chopped flat-leaf parsley
¼ teaspoon minced garlic
½ cup grated Parmesan cheese
½ cup olive oil
Salt
Freshly ground black pepper

1. In the bowl of a food processor combine the broccoli, parsley, garlic, and Parmesan and begin processing.
2. While the processor is running add the olive oil in a thin stream and blend until smooth. Add salt and pepper to taste.

NUTRITION FACTS

Serving Size: 1 serving ■ Servings Per Recipe: 8 ■ Amount Per Serving ■ Calories: 182 ■ Calories from fat: 155 (85% of tot cal) ■ % Daily Value* ■ Total Fat 17g 27% ■ Saturated Fat 4g 21% ■ Cholesterol 10mg 3% ■ Sodium 234mg 10% ■ Total Carbo 2g 1% ■ Dietary Fiber 1g 3% ■ Sugars 0g ■ Protein 6g ■ Vitamin A 51% ■ Vitamin C 50% ■ Calcium 20% ■ Iron 5%

*Percent Daily Values are based on a 2000 calorie diet. Your daily values may be higher or lower depending upon your caloric intake.

In Arkansas, a law requires schools to calculate body mass index for all students, and bans vending machines in elementary schools.

Vegetable Fajitas R

8 SERVINGS

Fajitas are a fun way to allow children some choice in putting together their meals. Consider adding chicken, beef, or shrimp to the marinade for variety. Other spring and summer vegetables such as asparagus, squash, or eggplant are also excellent choices for this recipe. Sauté the vegetables the night before, reheat in the morning, and send them to school in a vacuum bottle with the toppings like cheese and Guacamole (page 144) on the side. Bigger kids will love assembling their own fajitas at lunchtime.

3 tablespoons olive oil

1 tablespoon red wine vinegar

1/2 teaspoon whole cumin seed, toasted and ground

1 1/2 teaspoons kosher salt

1/2 teaspoon freshly ground black pepper

1 cup julienned red bell pepper (1 large)

1 cup julienned yellow bell pepper (1 large)

1 cup julienned zucchini (1 large)

1 cup julienned summer squash (1 large)

1 cup julienned carrots (1 to 2 large)

1 cup sliced yellow onion (1 large)

1 cup Roma tomatoes (3 large), seeded and diced

1 cup red onion (1 large), diced small

1 tablespoon lime juice

1 teaspoon seeded and chopped fresh jalapeño pepper (1 small)

1/2 cup chopped fresh cilantro

3 cloves garlic, chopped

8 6-inch flour tortillas

1. Combine oil, vinegar, cumin, ¾ teaspoon salt, and ¼ teaspoon ground pepper in a large bowl. Add the bell peppers, squashes, carrots, and yellow onion, and marinate in the refrigerator for 30 minutes.

2. Combine the tomatoes, red onion, lime juice, jalapeño, cilantro, garlic, and remaining salt and pepper to make a salsa.

3. In a large skillet, sauté the marinated vegetables until just soft.

4. Warm the tortillas. Serve with sautéed vegetables and salsa.

NUTRITION FACTS

Serving Size: 1 tortilla plus 1 cup vegetables ■ Servings Per Recipe: 8 ■ Amount Per Serving ■ Calories: 231 ■ Calories from fat: 69 (57% of tot cal) ■ % Daily Value* ■ Total Fat 8g 12% ■ Saturated Fat 1g 5% ■ Cholesterol 0mg 0% ■ Sodium 702mg 29% ■ Total Carbo 36g 12% ■ Dietary Fiber 3g 10% ■ Sugars 5g ■ Protein 6g ■ Vitamin A 581% ■ Vitamin C 184% ■ Calcium 14% ■ Iron 18%

*Percent Daily Values are based on a 2000 calorie diet. Your daily values may be higher or lower depending upon your caloric intake.

Corn and Black-eyed Pea Stew FC

8 SERVINGS

We love hearty soups and stews of all kinds, especially those made with beans and legumes. These filling ingredients not only taste great, but give warmth and energy in colder climes. Try variations by replacing the black-eyed peas with other types of beans like navy, cannellini, or even lima, and don't be afraid to add other vegetables like the many varieties of squash.

1 pound dried black-eyed peas
¾ cup Spanish onion (1 medium), diced small
¾ teaspoon minced garlic (1 clove)
2 teaspoons olive oil

¼ teaspoon ground cumin

⅛ teaspoon cayenne pepper

½ cup seeded and diced green bell pepper (1 small)

2 cups fresh corn kernels (about 2 large ears)

2 cups Roma tomatoes (4 to 5), seeded and diced

¾ teaspoon kosher salt

⅛ teaspoon freshly ground black pepper

Cooked brown rice, polenta (see page 131), or other grain

1. In a large stock pot bring 2 quarts of water to a simmer. Add the black-eyed peas and cook for 2 to 4 hours until the beans are soft. Add water while cooking as needed.
2. After the beans are fully cooked, drain them and set aside. Sauté the onion and garlic in the oil in a medium saucepan until translucent, about 2 minutes.
3. Add the cumin and cayenne and sauté for 1 minute.
4. Add the bell pepper and sauté 4 minutes.
5. Add the corn, cooked beans, tomatoes, salt, and pepper, and cook for 5 minutes more. Serve with cooked brown rice, polenta, or another grain of your choice.

NUTRITION FACTS

Serving Size: About 5.5 ounces ■ Servings Per Recipe: 8 ■ Amount Per Serving ■ Calories: 253 ■ Calories from fat: 23 (9% of tot cal) ■ % Daily Value* ■ Total Fat 3g 4% ■ Saturated Fat 0g 2% ■ Cholesterol 0mg 0% ■ Sodium 241mg 10% ■ Total Carbo 46g 15% ■ Dietary Fiber 8g 32% ■ Sugars 6g ■ Protein 15g ■ Vitamin A 48% Vitamin C 52%

*Percent Daily Values are based on a 2000 calorie diet. Your daily values may be higher or lower depending upon your caloric intake.

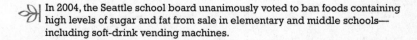

In 2004, the Seattle school board unanimously voted to ban foods containing high levels of sugar and fat from sale in elementary and middle schools—including soft-drink vending machines.

Sandwiches!

Almost every kid loves a good peanut butter or grilled cheese sandwich, but every day? Not only is it boring, but it doesn't encourage nutritional variety, which is key to a healthy diet. Rather than fill up pages with sandwich "recipes," we've opted to give you some sandwich suggestions:

Cashew or almond butter and honey on 12-grain bread

Add dried cranberries and walnuts to your favorite chicken salad

Stuff a salad in a pita (keep the dressing on the side if it's going in a lunch box)

Give them a Gobbler! Turkey, cranberry sauce, and a thin layer of mashed sweet potatoes or leftover stuffing

Grilled vegetables with goat cheese on toasted wholegrain bread make for a tasty and healthful combination

Grilled portabella mushroom with melted Swiss cheese, avocado, and honey mustard is a big hit with the older kids

Instead of the standard mayonnaise or mustard, use pepper jellies on ham, turkey, and chicken sandwiches

Skip the bread and use some Boston Bibb lettuce leaves as sandwich wrappers

How about a fruit sandwich? That might even make for an interesting new breakfast—slices of your favorite fruits between thin slices of our Banana Bread (page 119), for example.

Sit down with your kids and ask them to brainstorm sandwich ideas with you. You might be surprised by the combinations they come up with. One of our personal favorites was when a four-year-old put peanut butter and cheese in a sandwich and LOVED it. We're not saying it was healthy, but we admired the kid's sense of adventure, and as long as he has that he'll keep trying new things and broadening his palate, which ought to be a primary goal for every parent.

Vegetable Fried Rice FC

8 SERVINGS

Fried rice is an Asian specialty that is made from rice that has been cooked and refrigerated overnight before being fried with a variety of other ingredients. It's important to allow the rice to dry in the refrigerator overnight because it will have a better texture and greater intensity of flavor. The vegetables in this recipe aren't written in stone. Gather your family around the table the day before you plan on serving this and come up with your own vegetable combinations. Add meat, more eggs, or shrimp for a heartier meal.

> 3 cups brown rice, uncooked
>
> ¾ teaspoon minced garlic
>
> ¼ teaspoon grated fresh ginger
>
> 3 tablespoons vegetable oil
>
> 3 large eggs, beaten
>
> ¼ cup shredded carrots (1 small)
>
> ½ cup fresh green beans, sliced in ½-inch lengths
>
> ½ cup red bell peppers (1 small), diced small
>
> ¾ cup sliced mushrooms
>
> ½ cup shelled peas (about ½ pound in the pod)
>
> 2 tablespoons light soy sauce
>
> ¼ cup sliced scallions (green onions)

1. *The night before:* Bring 4 cups of water to a boil. Add the rice, reduce the heat to low, and cook until soft, approximately 40 minutes. Once the rice is tender and all the water absorbed, spread the

---

A company called Munchkin Bottling arranged to have the logos of Mountain Dew and Pepsi placed on baby bottles. Babies are four times more likely to consume soft drinks from these than standard bottles.

cooked rice on a cookie sheet and place in the refrigerator to dry uncovered overnight.

2. *The next day:* Stir-fry the garlic and ginger in a wok or large sauté pan with 2 tablespoons of the vegetable oil over medium heat, taking care not to burn them, about 1 minute.

3. Add the remaining tablespoon of oil and heat. Then add and scramble the eggs. Once the eggs are scrambled, add the rice and stir-fry until hot.

4. Add the vegetables, soy sauce, and scallions, and cook for 2 minutes, allowing the flavors to blend.

NUTRITION FACTS

Serving Size: 1 cup ■ Servings Per Recipe: 8 ■ Amount Per Serving ■ Calories: 183 ■ Calories from fat: 59 (32% of tot cal) ■ % Daily Value* ■ Total Fat 7g 10% ■ Saturated Fat 1g 7% ■ Cholesterol 92mg 31% ■ Sodium 238mg 10% ■ Total Carbo 25g 8% ■ Dietary Fiber 2g 8% ■ Sugars 1g ■ Protein 6g ■ Vitamin A 156% ■ Vitamin C 36% ■ Calcium 4% ■ Iron 13%

*Percent Daily Values are based on a 2000 calorie diet. Your daily values may be higher or lower depending upon your caloric intake.

Grilled Chicken Marinated with Yogurt and Asian Spices R

8 SERVINGS

Yogurt has a long tradition in Middle Eastern cuisine. It is used as a base for everything from condiments to sauces and marinades. In a marinade, it not only adds flavor, but it acts as a tenderizer. The flavors in this dish are robust, but they are tempered by the yogurt and are tremendously pleasing. Don't hesitate to put this in a lunch box as long as it is packed with a small ice pack.

Marinade

1½ cups plain nonfat yogurt

2 teaspoons minced garlic

¼ teaspoon whole cumin seed

¼ teaspoon curry powder

Pinch freshly ground black pepper

⅛ teaspoon yellow mustard seeds, ground

Pinch ground celery seeds

1 teaspoon minced fresh ginger

Pinch grated nutmeg

1½ teaspoons kosher salt

Sauce

3 tablespoons extra virgin olive oil

1 teaspoon minced garlic (1 clove)

¾ cup red onion (1 large), diced small

1 medium cucumber, peeled, seeded, and diced

Pinch curry powder

Freshly ground black pepper

Pinch whole cumin seeds

8 Roma tomatoes, chopped (1½ pounds)

Kosher salt

3 pounds boneless skinless chicken breasts

1. Combine all marinade ingredients and pour over the chicken in a nonreactive container. Allow to sit in the refrigerator for at least 1 hour, but it is best if you can marinate the chicken overnight.
2. To make the sauce: In a small bowl, combine the olive oil, garlic, onion, cucumber, curry, pepper, cumin, tomato, season with salt and pepper and set aside for 1 hour at room temperature.
3. Charbroil the chicken, top with sauce, and serve.

NUTRITION FACTS

Serving Size: 6 oz meat with sauce ■ Servings Per Recipe: 8 ■ Amount Per Serving ■ Calories: 390 ■ Calories from fat: 193 (49% of tot cal) ■ % Daily Value* ■ Total Fat 21g 33% ■ Saturated Fat 5g 35% ■

Cholesterol 110mg 37% ■ Sodium 591mg 25% ■ Total Carbo 9g 3% ■ Dietary Fiber 1g 5% ■ Sugars 9g ■ Protein 39g ■ Vitamin A 52% Vitamin C 43% ■ Calcium 14% Iron 1%

*Percent Daily Values are based on a 2000 calorie diet. Your daily values may be high or lower depending upon your caloric intake.

※

Shrimp Stir-Fry R

■

8 SERVINGS

Stir-frying is a quick and easy meal preparation. A hot wok or large skillet is a must, as is a plethora of fresh veggies. Replace the shrimp with scallops, chicken, or tofu for variation and serve with a side of brown rice.

2 tablespoons canola oil

2 tablespoons minced fresh ginger

1 tablespoon minced garlic (1 clove)

2 tablespoons sliced scallions (green onions)

2 pounds medium shrimp, peeled and deveined

1 cup thinly sliced celery (1 to 2 stalks)

1 cup julienned carrots (2 large)

1 cup julienned red onion (1 large)

½ cup julienned red bell peppers (1 medium)

½ cup blanched snap peas

½ cup oyster sauce

1 tablespoon sesame oil

2 tablespoons chopped cilantro

2 ounces fresh mung bean sprouts (about ½ cup)

1. In a wok, heat the oil and quickly stir-fry the ginger, garlic, and scallions.

2. Add the shrimp and stir-fry 3 to 4 minutes.
3. Add the celery, carrots, and onions and stir-fry for 2 minutes.
4. Add the pepper and snap peas and stir-fry another 2 minutes.
5. Add the oyster sauce and stir-fry 2 more minutes.
6. Add a drizzle of sesame oil to finish. Remove from heat and garnish with cilantro and bean sprouts.

NUTRITION FACTS

Serving Size: About 1½ cups ▪ Servings Per Recipe: 8 ▪ Amount Per Serving ▪ Calories: 235 ▪ Calories from fat: 99 (42% of tot cal) ▪ % Daily Value* ▪ Total Fat 11g 17% ▪ Saturated Fat 1g 6% ▪ Cholesterol 172mg 57% ▪ Sodium 496mg 21% ▪ Total Carbo 9g 3% ▪ Dietary Fiber 2g 8% ▪ Sugars 2g ▪ Protein 24g ▪ Vitamin A 533% ▪ Vitamin C 63% ▪ Calcium 10% ▪ Iron 34%

*Percent Daily Values are based on a 2000 calorie diet. Your daily values may be higher or lower depending upon your caloric intake.

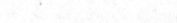

Butternut Squash Soup with Fried Sage Leaves CPF

8 SERVINGS

Butternut squash is a mainstay during the late summer and early fall season in New England. It can be prepared countless ways, but this soup is one of our favorites because it combines the sweetness of the squash with the perfume of the sage and the spiciness of cloves and herbs.

¼ cup extra virgin olive oil
16 whole fresh sage leaves, rinsed and dried

In an average gym class, a child is aerobically active for only 3.5 minutes.

4 large butternut squash, peeled, seeded, and roughly chopped

1 beet, peeled and roughly chopped

1 onion, roughly chopped

5 large carrots, sliced

4 stalks celery, chopped

¼ cup minced flat-leaf parsley

6 cloves garlic, minced

1 teaspoon minced fresh thyme,

2 quarts vegetable stock

1 teaspoon kosher salt

⅛ teaspoon freshly ground black pepper

1. In a medium stockpot over medium heat, heat the oil and fry the sage leaves until crisp, about 45 seconds. Remove them from the oil and reserve.
2. In the same pot, sauté the squash, beet, onion, carrots, and celery for 10 minutes.
3. Stir in the parsley, garlic, and thyme, and cook for 5 more minutes.
4. Add the vegetable stock, cover, and simmer 5 minutes until all of the vegetables are tender.
5. Add the salt and pepper to taste, and adjust as needed.
6. Puree with a hand blender.
7. Serve hot, garnished with fried sage leaves.

NUTRITION FACTS

Serving Size: 1 cup ▪ Servings Per Recipe: 8 ▪ Amount Per Serving ▪ Calories: 254 ▪ Calories from fat: 67 (26% of tot cal) ▪ % Daily Value* ▪ Total Fat 7g 11% ▪ Saturated Fat 1g 5% ▪ Cholesterol 0mg 0% ▪ Sodium 428mg 18% ▪ Total Carbo 47g 16% ▪ Dietary Fiber 9g 37% ▪ Sugars 9g ▪ Protein 5g ▪ Vitamin A 3282% ▪ Vitamin C 113% ▪ Calcium 18% ▪ Iron 34%

*Percent Daily Values are based on a 2000 calorie diet. Your daily values may be higher or lower depending upon your caloric intake.

Resource Guide

NAME	URL	CATEGORY	COMMENT
American Farmland Trust	www.farmland.org	Farming	Conserving Farmland
Berkeley Unified School District	www.berkeley.k12.ca.us	School Food	
Beyond Pesticides	www.beyondpesticides.org	Sustainable Food	
Big Oven Recipe Software	www.bigoven.com	Recipe Software	
Bioneers	www.bioneers.org	Environmental Activism	
Blue Ocean Institute	www.blueocean.org/seafood	Sustainable Seafood	
Center for Disease Control and Prevention	www.cdc.gov	Government/ Health	
Center for Ecoliteracy	www.ecoliteracy.org	School Food/ Wellness	Rethinking School Lunch Wellness Guide
Center for Environmental Health	www.cehca.org	Environment	
Center for Science in the Public Interest	www.cspinet.org	Sustainable Environment	
Chef Ann Cooper	www.chefann.com www.lunchlessons.org	School Food/ Sustainable Food	Ann's sites
Chef's Collaborative	www.chefscollaborative.org	Sustainable food/ agriculture	
Chez Panisse Foundation	www.chezpanissefoundation.org	School Food/ Education	Edible School Yard
Chipotle Grill	www.chipotle.com	Healthy Fast Food	
Cloud Institute for Sustainability Education	www.sustainabilityed.org	Sustainability Education	
Community Alliance with Family Farmers	www.caff.org	Sustainable Agriculture	
Community Food Security Coalition	www.foodsecurity.org	Food Security/ Hunger Relief	
Composters	www.composters.com	Composting	
Consumer's Union Eco-Labels	www.eco-labels.org	Shopping	
Container Gardening	www.gardenguides.com	Gardening	

NAME	URL	CATEGORY	COMMENT
Cook's Garden	www.cooksgarden.com	Gardening	
Coop America	www.coopamerica.org	Sustainable Shopping	
Earth 911	www.earth911.org	Recycling	
Earthpledge	www.earthpledge.com	Farming/ Environment	Hosts Farm to Table
Eat Well Guide	www.eatwellguide.org	Sustainable Meat & Poultry	
Edible School Yard	www.edibleschoolyard.org	School Food/ Gardens	Hosted by Chez Panisse Foundation
EECO Farm	www.eecofarm.org	Gardening	
Environmental Defense	www.edf.org	Environment	
Farm to School National Site	www.farmtoschool.org	Farm to School Programs	
Farm to Table	www.farmtotable.org	Farming	Earthpledge
Field to Plate	www.fieldtoplate.com	Food/Farming	
Feingold Association	www.feingold.org	ADHD and Food	
Food project	www.thefoodproject.org	Food/Farming	
Food Routes	www.foodroutes.org	Food/Farming/ Education	
Food Time Line	www.foodtimeline.org	Food Education	
FoodChange	www.foodchange.org	School Food	CookShop/ School Food Plus
FullBloom Baking Company	www.fullbloom.com	Healthy Food Service	
Green Guide	www.thegreenguide.com	Green Shopping	
Happy D Ranch	www.happydranch.com/	Worm Farming	
Harlem Children's Zone	www.hcz.org	School Food	
Harvard School of Health	www.hsph.harvard.edu/ nutritionsource	Healthy Public Nutrition	
Johnny's Seeds	www.johnnyseeds.com	Gardening	
Just Food	www.justfood.org	Food/Farming	
Kellogg Foundation	www.wkkf.org	Foundation	Food & Society Policy Fellows Supports numerous NGOs
Kids Gardening	www.kidsgardening.com	Gardening	
Laptop Lunches	www.laptoplunches.com	Lunch Boxes	
Leopold Center	www.leopold.iastate.edu	Sustainable Agriculture	
Local Harvest	www.localharvest.org	Food/Farming	

NAME	URL	CATEGORY	COMMENT
Monterey Bay Aquarium	www.mbayaq.org	Sustainable Seafood	
National Campaign for Sustainable Agriculture	www.sustainableagriculture.net	Sustainable Agriculture	
National Green Pages	www.greenpages.org	Shopping	
National Resources Defense Council	www.nrdc.org	Environment	
National School Lunch Program	www.fns.usda.gov/cnd/Lunch/default.htm	Government/Policy	USDA site
Natural Ovens	www.naturalovens.com	School Food	Appleton, WI
Nature Conservancy	www.nature.org	Land Conservation	
New York Coalition for Healthy School Lunches (NYCHSL)	www.healthylunches.org	School Food	
Northeast Organic Farming Association	www.nofa.org	Organic Farming	
O'Naturals	www.onaturals.com	Healthy Fast Food	
Ocean Arks	www.oceanarks.org	Sustainable Ecology	
Organic Consumers Association	www.organicconsumers.org	Organics	
Organic Farming Research Foundation	www.ofrf.org	Organic Farming	
Organic Trade Association	www.ota.com	Organics	
Pesticide Action Network	www.panna.org	Pesticides	
Quail Hill Farm	www.peconiclandtrust.org	Farming/CSA	
Ross Institute	www.rossinstitute.org	Education	
Ross School	www.ross.org	School Food	
School Lunch Initiative	www.schoollunchinitiative.org	School Food/Education	
Seeds of Change	www.seedsofchange.com	Gardening	
Slow Food USA	www.slowfoodusa.org	School Food	Slow in Schools Wellness Guide
Spoons Across America	www.spoonsacrossamerica.org	Childhood Culinary Education	Supported by the Beard Foundation
Stonyfield Yogurt	www.stonyfield.com	Healthy School Vending Machines	

NAME	URL	CATEGORY	COMMENT
Supersize Me	www.supersizeme.com	Obesity and Fast Food	Educational content
Union of Concerned Scientists	www.ucsaction.org	Environment	
USDA Child Nutrition Services	www.fns.usda.gov/cnd	School Food	
Worldwatch Institute	www.worldwatch.org	Environment	
Yale Sustainable Food Project	www.yale.edu/sustainablefood	Food/Education	Alice Waters—founder

The Center for Ecoliteracy's Model Wellness Policy Guide*

The Center for Ecoliteracy, in collaboration with Slow Food USA and the Chez Panisse Foundation, has prepared this Model Wellness Policy Guide. The Guide provides language and instructions for drafting a Wellness Policy that places health at the center of the academic curriculum.

Compiled and produced by Janet Brown, program officer for Food Systems, Center for Ecoliteracy.

ACKNOWLEDGMENTS

The partners in this endeavor gratefully acknowledge the following experts who reviewed this document, and through their expertise, improved it.

Eleanor Bertino, Publicist, Eleanor Bertino Public Relations
Karen Brown, Designer, Karen Brown Design
Ann Cooper, Author and Chef

*Reprinted in its entirety from the Center for Ecoliteracy, www.ecoliteracy.org/programs/wellness_policy.html

Ann M. Evans, Nutrition Education Consultant, California
   Department of Education
Joan Dye Gussow, Mary Swartz Rose Professor Emeritus of
   Nutrition and Education, Teachers College, Columbia
   University
Brian Halweil, Senior Researcher, Worldwatch Institute
Marion Nestle, Paulette Goddard Professor of Nutrition, Food
   Studies, and Public Health, New York University
Margo Wootan, Director of Nutrition Policy, Center for
   Science in the Public Interest

The Guide is inspired by the work of the Child Nutrition Advisory Council of the Berkeley Unified School District. That working group, a forerunner of the Wellness Committee, drafted and supported to adoption the first school district wellness policy of its kind in the nation in August of 1999. Their inspirational language is an integrator throughout the Guide that ensures that the intention in adopting the policy, and the policy itself, remain connected.

THE FEDERAL GOVERNMENT has issued a mandate, through the Child Nutrition and WIC Reauthorization Act of 2004, that provides us all with a great opportunity: to establish standards for diet and health in our nation's public schools. The Wellness Policy process calls for each school district to form a Wellness Committee and draft a district Wellness Policy that addresses the quality of meals served at school, regularity of physical education, and instruction connected to diet and health. These school Wellness Policies will go into effect at the beginning of the school year in 2006. The Center for Ecoliteracy in collaboration with Slow Food USA and the Chez Panisse Foundation hope you will join us in this exciting endeavor by participating on a Wellness Committee at your neighborhood school, and recruiting others to serve.

The first step is to call your school district and determine the status of your local Wellness Committee. Wellness Committees are intended to be diverse, inclusive, and representative of the local community they serve. In addition to joining, or acting as an advisor to someone already on the committee, you may also be instrumental in bringing others to the process, insuring greater diversity.

Here are some basic principles on which we can all agree:

- Healthy children are the foundation of a healthy society;
- Healthy, well-nourished children are better able to learn;
- All children deserve nutritious, safe, and deliciously prepared food;
- Eating habits developed in childhood will affect health throughout life;
- Knowledge of food—how it is grown, who grows it, how it is prepared, its connection to tradition, and its influence in shaping the future of society—is integral to a healthy education.

The Wellness Policy development process provides us all with an opportunity to put these values-based principles into practice. In that spirit, the Center for Ecoliteracy, in collaboration with Slow Food USA and the Chez Panisse Foundation, has developed a Model Wellness Policy Guide based on the groundbreaking work of the Berkeley Unified School District's Wellness Committee, formerly known as the Child Nutrition Advisory Council. The brilliance, determination, and foresight of this pioneer group led to the formulation of the first public school district food policy of its kind in the nation. That policy has been emulated by school districts across the nation, has influenced the current Wellness Policy process, and is acknowledged as the foundation for Grab Five, the national school meal policy of the United Kingdom.

Given the rapid rise in childhood obesity and diabetes, we now have no choice but to change school food policy on a national level. Join us in this extraordinary opportunity to influence the development of school district policies that promote human and environmental health, high academic achievement, and a sustainable future.

How to Use This Guide

- The Model Wellness Policy Guide (the Guide) provides recommendations and model language for development of a comprehensive school Wellness Policy.
- The Guide is structured in numbered sections that correspond to the minimum requirements of the Child Nutrition and WIC Reauthorization Act of 2004.
- You must set goals as required by the Act. Model language and recommendations are provided by Center for Ecoliteracy, Slow Food USA, and the Chez Panisse Foundation to assist you in developing a comprehensive Wellness Policy that sets high standards for healthy learning. The Guide includes narrative language under headings and sub-headings that make clear the district's motivation in enacting policy, and specific language for individual policy points. You may use the language exactly as is, or adapt it to fit your school's unique culture and needs.
- Instructions throughout this guide will appear in *italics*.

Background

In the Child Nutrition and WIC Reauthorization Act of 2004, the U.S. Congress established a requirement that all school districts with a federally funded school meal program form a Wellness Committee to draft a Wellness Policy by the start of the 2006–2007 school year. The law requires that these policies must, at a minimum:

1. Include goals for nutrition education, physical activity, and other school-based activities that promote student wellness.
2. Establish nutrition guidelines for all foods available on cam-

pus during the school day with the objectives of promoting student health and reducing childhood obesity.

3. Provide assurance that guidelines for reimbursable school meals shall not be less restrictive than regulations and guidance issued by the Secretary of Agriculture.

4. Establish a plan for measuring the impact and implementation of the local wellness policy.

5. Involve parents, students, and representatives of the school authority, school board, school administrators, and the public, in development of the local Wellness Policy.

Your commitment to the Wellness Policy development process will ensure that a complete understanding of wellness includes additional enrichment and learning opportunities for the whole child that:

- Integrate core curriculum with learning experiences in instructional gardens, kitchen classrooms, cafeterias, and local farms;
- Build skills linked to meal preparation;
- Emphasize fresh, local, seasonal, whole, and sustainably grown foods from local sources;
- Model recycling, reduction, and composting of waste;
- Develop positive social interactions, good manners, and enjoyment of meals through positive dining experiences;
- Lead to a basic understanding of the principles of sustainability;
- Enhance respect for cultural and agricultural values;
- Include families and the community as a resource in the learning process.

Developing an Opening Statement

School Wellness Policies are a direct expression of local care and concern for the well-being of young people. The best policies reflect core community values and culture, regional tastes and food traditions, and an emphasis on learning outcomes connected to diet, health, and environmental education.

*Many school districts begin their Wellness Policies with a visionary **statement of responsibility** and a **preamble** that sets forth the conditions defining the need to act. This statement contains the vision of the school district and community for its students. This shared vision is the foundation of a partnership between school and community that makes clear the school district's intention in adopting the policy and leads to realization of policy goals.*

In drafting a Wellness Policy for your school district, you may use the following sample language as is, or adapt it to fit your district's unique circumstances and needs.

Sample Statement of Responsibility

The Board of Education recognizes that there is a link between nutrition education, the food served in schools, physical activity, and environmental education, and that wellness is affected by all of these. The Board also recognizes the important connection between a healthy diet and a student's ability to learn effectively and achieve high standards in school.

The Board recognizes that it is the District's role, as part of the larger community, to model and actively practice, through policies and procedures: the promotion of family health, physical activity, good nutrition, sustainable agriculture, and environmental restoration.

The Board of Education further recognizes that the sharing and enjoyment of food, and participation in physical activities, are fundamental experiences for all people and are a primary way to nurture and celebrate our cultural diversity. These fundamental human experiences are vital bridges for building friendships, forming inter-generational bonds, and strengthening communities.

Sample Preamble

Wellness Policies often begin with a Preamble of statements that form the conceptual framework for change. The following are examples of such statements for consideration:

- Whereas, a healthy diet is connected to a student's ability to learn effectively and achieve high standards in school;
- Whereas, each day, students and their parents trust that the foods offered at school are wholesome and safe, and that the Governing Board is responsible for ensuring the safety of foods provided at school;
- Whereas, fresh, seasonal, local, sustainably grown foods are a primary and recommended source of nutrition for growing children, and pre-packaged, highly processed foods create a solid waste packaging management problem and expense for school districts;
- Whereas, small and mid-size farms and America's rural communities are under economic stress, and the public dollars from farm-to-school programs create a steady and reliable source of income for farmers;
- Whereas, the knowledge and skill-base for farming, gardening, food preservation, cooking, and the ritual of the table are disappearing from American life;
- Whereas, public school is an excellent place to nurture and preserve America's food traditions through storytelling, recipe swapping, rediscovering foodways, cooking classes, garden- and farm-based learning experiences, food served in the cafeteria, and connections to the core curriculum of science, math, language arts, history, geography, and social studies.

Wellness Policy Requirement 1

Set goals for nutrition education, physical activity, and other school-based activities that promote student wellness.

This required policy section provides language to address school-based activities that promote student wellness in the areas of **nutrition education, physical activity, and school-based learning experiences.**

You may use the language as is, or adapt it to fit your specific circumstances.

Nutrition Education

To help ensure the health and well being of each student attending—_____School District, and to provide guidance to school personnel in the areas of nutrition, health, physical activity and food service, the Governing Board encourages teachers, principals, and Nutrition Services employees to recognize the lunch period as an integral part of the educational program of the district, and work to implement the goals of this policy. The Governing Board will ensure that:

- No student in the_____School District goes hungry during school;
- An economically sustainable meal program makes available a healthy and nutritious breakfast, lunch, and after-school snack to every student at every school so that students are prepared to learn to their fullest potential;
- Each school in the district shall establish an instructional garden (tilled ground, raised bed, container, nearby park, community garden, farm, or lot), of sufficient size to provide students with experiences in planting, harvesting, preparation, serving, and tasting foods, including ceremonies and celebrations that observe food traditions, integrated with

nutrition education and core curriculum, and articulated with state standards;

- Staff shall integrate hands-on experiences in gardens and kitchen classrooms, and enriched activities such as farm field studies, farmers' markets tours, and visits to community gardens, with core curriculum so that students begin to understand how food reaches the table and the implications that has for their health and future;
- Sampling and tasting in school gardens and kitchen classrooms shall be encouraged as part of nutrition education;
- Staff is encouraged to utilize food from school gardens and local farms in kitchen classrooms and cafeterias based upon availability and acceptability;
- Schools shall use food as an integrator and central focus of education about human events, history, and celebrations, and shall encourage classes to use food and cooking as part of a learning experience that sheds light on the customs, history, traditions, and cuisine of various countries and cultures;
- Eating experiences, gardens, cooking classes, and nutrition education are integrated into the core academic curriculum at all grade levels;
- Schools shall promote food-centered activities that are healthful, enjoyable, developmentally appropriate, culturally relevant, and participatory, such as contests, promotions, taste testing, farm visits, school gardens, and kitchen classrooms;
- Lunch periods shall be scheduled so that students do not have to eat lunch unusually early or late, and ideally, so that they come after periods of exercise;
- All school eating areas shall contain free, safe, drinking water sources and facilities for washing hands;
- At each school site, students shall play a role in a recycling program that begins with the purchase of recycled products

and maximizes the reduction of waste by recycling, reusing, composting, and purchasing recycled products;
- Meals will be attractively presented and served in a pleasant environment with sufficient time for eating, while fostering good eating habits, enjoyment of meals, good manners, and respect for others;
- Students at the K–8 level will not be involved in the sale of candy, sodas, cookies and sweets at any school sponsored event or for any fundraising activity;
- A full-service kitchen will be installed at school sites where public bond money is expended to repair or remodel a school;
- The Maintenance Committee shall include kitchen facilities, food preparation and storage of equipment as a high priority in its comprehensive maintenance policy;
- Food Services shall work to modernize computer equipment and programs, and institute an automated accounting system and card swipe system to protect student privacy.

Physical Activity

The Governing Board recognizes the positive benefits of physical activity for student health and academic achievement. Recognizing that physical education is a crucial and integral part of a child's education, the District will provide opportunities to ensure that students engage in healthful levels of vigorous physical activity to promote and develop the student's physical, mental, emotional, and social well-being. Besides promoting high levels of personal achievement and a positive self-image, physical education activities should teach students how to cooperate in the achievement of common goals.

The components of the District's physical education program shall include a variety of kinesthetic activities, including team, individual, and cooperative sports and physical activities, as well as aesthetic movement forms, such as dance, yoga or the martial arts. Students shall be given opportunities for physical activity through a range of before- and/or after-school programs including, but not limited to, intramurals, interscholastic athletics, and physical activity clubs. The Governing Board will ensure that:

- Physical education teachers shall develop and implement a curriculum that connects and demonstrates the inter-relationship between physical activity, good nutrition, and health;
- The District shall enhance the quality of physical education curricula and increase training of physical education teachers through site-based and district-wide staff development;
- Students shall have opportunities to enjoy physical activity through participation in gardening programs;
- An appropriate alternative activity shall be provided for students with a physical disability that may restrict excessive physical exertion;
- Physical education staff shall appropriately limit the amount or type of physical exercise required of students during air pollution episodes, excessively hot weather, or other inclement conditions.

Physical Activity Exemptions

The Superintendent or designee may grant temporary exemption from physical education under any of the following conditions:

- The student is ill or injured and a modified program to meet his/her needs cannot be provided;
- The student is enrolled for one-half-time or less;
- A student in grades 10–12 attends a regional occupational center or program and attendance in physical education

courses results in hardship because of the travel time
involved;
- A high school student is engaged in a regular school-
sponsored interscholastic athletic program carried on wholly
or partially after regular school hours;
- A student is either:

  - Age 16 years or older and has been enrolled in grade 10
    for one or more academic years;
  - Enrolled as a postgraduate student;
  - Enrolled in a juvenile home, ranch, camp, or forestry
    camp school with scheduled recreation and exercise.

School-Based Learning Experiences

The Governing Board recognizes that experiential learning activities
that assist students to make connections between diet, health, and environment are critical to formation of student understanding of personal wellness within a larger context of environmental health.
Schools play a crucial role in educating students on environmental issues and preparing them to be the stewards of their natural resources.
The quality of life in future generations will depend upon our students'
willingness and ability to solve today's environmental problems and
prevent new ones from developing.

The Governing Board desires to offer environmental education
that fosters attitudes of personal responsibility toward the environment and provides students with the concepts, knowledge, and skills
needed to contribute meaningfully to decisions involving the environment and its resources. At all grade levels, the Governing Board urges
that environmental facts should be taught as they relate to each other,
so that students will understand basic ecological principles and appreciate the interrelated nature of living processes, the effect of human
activities on ecological relationships, and the interdependence of hu-
manity and nature.

The Governing Board also recognizes that interactive hands-on experiences with the natural world can empower students to actively investigate the ecological principles that sustain our environment. Through the use of experiential learning opportunities in school gardens and cooking classes, students can better understand where their food comes from and how the food choices they and their families make impact the health of the larger social and natural communities within which they live. The Governing Board will ensure that:

- Staff is encouraged to integrate garden, nutrition education, cooking and eating experiences, and energy and renewable energy experiences into the curriculum for math, science, social studies, and language arts at all grade levels;
- Staff is encouraged to establish relationships with local farms so that farmers and farm workers will visit school classrooms and students will visit farms;
- Students are encouraged to recycle, conserve materials, water, and energy, use biodegradable materials when possible, and dispose of wastes in an environmentally sound way at school, in the cafeteria, in the school garden and kitchen classroom, and in all classroom-based activities;
- Food service and teaching staff shall work cooperatively to integrate experiences in cafeterias, instructional gardens, kitchen classrooms, and farm field trips with the formal learning experience of all students;
- School food service staff will work with school departments, and with community partners and the School Health Council, to facilitate student understanding and appreciation of fresh, local, sustainably grown food;
- Students shall be offered the opportunity to participate in outdoor education programs that make connections between diet, health, and the environment, and the interdependence of living things.

Professional Development

The Governing Board recognizes that using the local food system as a context for learning, and embedding nutrition education in a school's curriculum, generates new content for students to learn. It also requires teachers to learn new content and new strategies for teaching it. For good service personnel, new menus require new ways of purchasing, preparing, and presenting foods. The transition to an educational model that makes food and health central parts of the academic curriculum requires professional development. The Governing Board will ensure that:

- Regular professional development will be provided to enable the Food Service Staff to become full partners in providing excellent school meals;
- Regular professional development will be provided, at least annually, to teachers and the Food Service Staff on basic nutrition, nutrition education, and benefits of sustainable agriculture;
- Child Nutrition Services will be provided with USDA-approved computer software, training, and support to implement nutrient-based menu planning when such flexibility is desirable;
- Child Nutrition Services Staff and district teachers will receive professional development jointly, at least once a year, to facilitate a more coordinated approach to integrating classroom lessons with experiences in gardens, kitchen classrooms, and the cafeteria.

Waste Reduction

The Board recognizes that school meal programs that utilize pre-packaged, processed foods consistently generate more solid waste than those that are cooked from whole ingredients. A shift to cooking meals from fresh, whole ingredients usually leads to a reduction in solid waste, and in the expense associated with waste disposal. The Governing Board will ensure that:

- Meals prepared at school utilize fresh, whole, unpackaged, unprocessed or minimally processed ingredients, to the maximum extent possible, in order to preserve nutritional content and reduce packaging waste;
- Cafeterias model environmentally sound practices, educate and involve students and staff in reducing waste, composting, recycling and purchasing recycled material;
- Post consumer food waste is composted and returned for use in the school garden program;
- Packaging containing school meals is made of recycled content and should be recycled;
- Savings from waste reduction policies administered by the school are tracked, and those savings are rebated to the school site for use in furthering the waste reduction and garden-based learning program.

Wellness Policy Requirement 2

Establish nutrition guidelines for all foods available on campus during the school day.

*This required policy section provides language to **establish nutrition guidelines** for all foods available on campus during the formal learning day. You may use the language as is, or adapt it to fit your specific circumstances.*

Part of the educational mission of the_____School District is to improve the health of the entire community by teaching students and families ways to establish and maintain life-long healthy eating habits. The mission shall be accomplished through nutrition education, physical education, garden-based learning experiences, environmental restoration, core academic content in the classroom, and the food served in schools. The Governing Board will ensure that:

- All qualified children will become eligible for free meals, through frequent checking and coordination with county social services;
- Maximum participation in the school meal program will be achieved by developing a coordinated, comprehensive outreach and promotion plan, and by putting systems in place that ensure the elimination of the stigma of accepting "free" lunch (such as a card swipe system);
- A shift from food-based planning to nutrient-based planning (as set forth in USDA guidelines) will be considered when it allows for more flexible food selection;
- The nutritional value of the food served will significantly improve upon USDA Dietary Guidelines through provision of nutritious, fresh, tasty, locally grown food that reflects community and cultural diversity;
- The reduced-price category for school lunch, breakfast, and snacks will be eliminated, so that all low-income children have healthy food available at no cost;
- Schools will provide students with at least 20 minutes to eat after sitting down for breakfast and 30–45 minutes after sitting down for lunch;
- Students will be encouraged to share food, as food sharing is a fundamental experience for all peoples. Despite concerns about allergies and other restrictions on some children's diets that can cause schools to discourage students from trading foods or beverages with classmates, sharing can be encouraged through service styles in the cafeteria, such as "family style," that provide students with the opportunity to serve themselves

from a common platter, and to pass platters of food to
tablemates;

- The Nutrition Services Director will develop and implement
a plan to support local sustainable agriculture by integrating
organic foods, as defined by the USDA National Organic
Program, into the meals served to students based on
availability and acceptability;
- Child Nutrition Services will coordinate its menus with
seasonal production of local farms, and with production in
school gardens, so that school meals will reflect seasonality
and local agriculture;
- Neighboring school districts will work cooperatively, and
whenever possible, purchase collectively, in order to increase
the amount of products purchased from local farms;
- Schools shall develop a "Healthy Snacks" and "Healthy
Parties" policy, and provide parents and teachers with a list
of healthy, affordable food choices for snacks and parties;
- Food offered to students and employees of the District during
the day as a snack, an incentive, or in school offices, whether
provided by parents or staff, shall be consistent with the
goals of the policy;
- Schools shall limit celebrations that involve food during the
school day to shared monthly birthday celebrations, and
should discourage serving foods and beverages that do not
meet nutrition standards for foods and beverages sold
individually;
- The foods used during classes as part of the learning process,
for fundraisers that take place at school, for at-school parties,
or school-sponsored events, should follow the nutrition

 Overweight is the most common and costly nutritional disorder of the
twenty-first century, affecting more than 1 billion adults and hundreds of
millions of children.

guidelines for snacks at school, and should be healthy, safe, and delicious;

- Parents and staff are encouraged to provide party snacks that are consistent with the goals of the policy, and to see to it that such items are served after the lunch hour whenever possible;

- Foods served at school will carry sufficient nutrition information to allow parents and students to make informed dietary choices. Information must clearly indicate dietary appropriateness such as vegetarian, vegan, or kosher, and include processes such as organically grown, irradiated, contains bovine growth hormone (rBGH), or has been genetically modified;

- The exposure of children to potentially harmful residues of toxic agricultural chemicals such as pesticides, herbicides, fertilizers, waxes, and fungicides will be reduced and/or eliminated by increasing the purchase of foods that are grown sustainably, without the use of toxic chemicals;

- Foods exposed to potentially harmful food additives and processes, such as bovine growth hormone, irradiation, high fructose corn syrup, excessive salt, artificial flavors and colors, hydrogenated oils (trans fats), preservatives, and genetic modification, shall be reduced and/or eliminated;

- Schools shall offer a variety of fresh fruits and vegetables, at least two non-fried vegetables and two fruit choices each day, and five different fruits and five different vegetables over the course of a week;

- No unhealthy food or beverage item may be advertised on school grounds, and fast food and "branded" food items shall not be offered for sale as part of any school meal program or as à la carte items;

- All revenue accrued by schools from foods sold on school campuses shall be spent only on school food services;

- Elementary schools shall not have vending machines or school stores accessible by students;
- Vending machines and school stores shall only offer approved items;
- Draft food and beverage vending contracts shall be made available to the public for inspection and comments before being signed by the District, and neither the District nor individual schools may sign exclusive contracts, or contracts with confidential clauses, with soft drink, fast food, or snack food companies.

Wellness Policy Requirement 3

Assure that guidelines for school meals are not less restrictive than those set at the federal level by the Secretary of Agriculture.

This required policy section provides language to assure that **guidelines for school meals set by the District Wellness Policy are not LESS restrictive than those set at the federal level by the Secretary of Agriculture.**

You may use the language as is, or adapt it to fit your specific circumstances.

- The Child Nutrition Services Director will review this policy and ensure that the policies are not less restrictive than those set by the Secretary of Agriculture or state law.

Wellness Policy Requirement 4

Establish a plan for measuring the impact and implementation of the local wellness policy.

This required policy section provides language to **establish a plan for** *measuring the impact and implementation of the local Wellness Policy.*

You may use the language as is, or adapt it to fit your specific circumstances.

The Wellness Committee is a working group of the school district instrumental in drafting the Wellness Policy and in facilitating its adoption by the Governing Board. Wellness Committees, School Health Councils, or Child Nutrition Advisory Councils (CNAC), are diverse and inclusive bodies that draft and review District wellness and nutrition policies and practices, track implementation, and recommend changes or improvements to the district. The Committee is responsible for addressing food-related topics of concern to the school community, and making Wellness Policy recommendations to the Board of Education.

In conjunction with adoption of a District Wellness Policy, the District shall establish a standing Wellness Committee, or School Health Council, to remain actively engaged with food service in monitoring the implementation of the Wellness Policy and in presenting recommendations to the Governing Board. The following guidelines pertain to the duties and responsibilities of standing Wellness Committees and food service to work cooperatively in evaluating success.

The standing Wellness Committe shall present to the Governing Board an Annual Report each year on the status of meeting the Wellness Policy goals. The report shall:

- Contain a review and comment on the Director's Annual Report, Profit and Loss Statement, Marketing Plan and Business Plan;
- Contain recommendations for improving the delivery and cost effectiveness of food services;
- Assist the Director of Child Nutrition Services in the development and implementation of the Outreach and Promotion Marketing plan;

- Recommend to the Governing Board strategies to eliminate potentially harmful food additives and processes, and to increase the amount of fresh, local produce offered through the School Meal Program;
- Make periodic reports, as the School Health Council deems necessary;
- Establish rules for decision-making;
- Ensure that the full complement of students, as specified in the policy, is represented on the School Health Council;
- Solicit student preferences through taste tests, surveys, and interviews, and through student participation on the district Wellness Committee.

Nutrition Services Annual Report

In order for the community to become full partners in the reinvention of food service, and in order for the Wellness Committee to be fully informed about food service function, and able to assess the impact and implementation of the local Wellness Policy, full transparency of food service operations and financials is necessary.

The board shall require, and each year Child Nutrition Services shall prepare, the Director's Annual Report for the Board of Education, which will include:

- Description of the level of service for each site and level of participation;
- Profit and Loss Statement for the past fiscal year;
- Outreach and Promotion Marketing Plan (with assistance from School Health Council);
- Budget for the future year;
- Report on the progress in meeting the Wellness Policy goals;
- Nutritional quality of the food being served;
- Inventory of equipment;

- Budget for maintenance and replacement equipment;
- Accounting of Child Nutrition Services' financial reserve, if any, and a budget allocating the reserve;
- Annual review of school food sales to determine:

  - Percentage of food purchased from local sources and the total dollar amount spent on local food;
  - Income benefit or less due to increases in local purchasing;
  - Opportunities to increase purchase of local and seasonal items;
  - Impacts on participation, and on fruit and vegetable consumption;
  - Degree of nutrition education students are receiving and how it is administered.

Such report shall inform the work of the Wellness Committee, which shall prepare an annual report to the Board of Education that contains a review and comment on the Director's Annual Report. The school district's Wellness Policy, Director's Annual Report, the Wellness Committee's Annual Report, and Monthly Menus shall be available at the District Office and on the Board of Education's website.

Public Policy

The School Board will work cooperatively with School Boards throughout the state and the nation to advance goals of wellness by:

- Advocating for label disclosure through State and Federal legislation that will clearly label food products that have been irradiated, genetically modified or have been exposed to bovine growth hormones;

- Sending a Board of Education resolution requesting support for labeling legislation to:

  - School Boards in the State;
  - State School Boards Association;
  - National School Boards Association.

Wellness Policy Requirement 5

Involve parents, students, and representatives of the school authority, the school board, school administrators, and the public, in development of the local Wellness Policy.

This required policy section provides language for **establishment of an inclusive process to develop a district Wellness Policy.**

You may use the language as is, or adapt it to fit your specific circumstances.

Wellness Committees are intended to be diverse and inclusive bodies, representative of the communities they serve. The membership should be large enough to ensure complete representation—cultural, ethnic, and economic— of the District, and manageable enough to be effective at conducting meetings and making decisions.

All of the stakeholders—school administrators, educators, food service personnel, and parents—are concerned with student health and academic performance and want to help schools make a more positive impact in this area. The District Wellness Policy spells out challenges to student wellness and proposes solutions that have been arrived at through an inclusive public process.

The school district should also develop a vehicle whereby all members of the community who wish to have input to the Wellness Policy development process, whether or not they participate on the Committee, can register their concerns and recommendations with the District.

When constituting a Wellness Committee, it is critically important that all sectors of the learning community that will be charged with implementing the

policy are represented including administration, food service, finance, facilities, communications, waste management, and instruction.

In addition, community members including parents, grandparents, farmers, school nurses, nutritionists, and health care professionals, and local organizations and agencies including community foundations, public health
departments, and local elected officials concerned with the health and well being of school age children are critically important contributors.

Experience has shown that innovation that occurs at a single school is unlikely to become part of lasting, District-wide change unless the innovation is
institutionalized in a District food policy. Innovations that are not supported
by all stakeholders have little chance of success.

Shared leadership creates the conditions for real and lasting change. Developing a school district Wellness Policy is a practical way to create a shared
vision and language about needed change. When the Board of Education
adopts a District Wellness Policy, the entire community knows the District is
committed to improving the school environment for children and youth, particularly the school food system.

Establishing a Wellness Committee

The Wellness Committee is a working group of the school district, instrumental in drafting the Wellness Policy. The Wellness Committee is responsible for
addressing food-related topics of concern to the school community and making Wellness Policy recommendations to the Board of Education.

The Board shall initiate a process to establish a Wellness Committee as a working group of the District. The Wellness Committee shall
draft a Wellness Policy and facilitate its adoption by the Governing
Board. The process to form the Wellness Committee shall be openly
announced, accessible, equitable, and inclusive. The Wellness Committee shall be a diverse and inclusive working group, representative of
the demographics of the school district as a whole.

The following guidelines pertain to the establishment of Wellness
Committees.

The recommended membership of the working group shall be as follows:

- The Superintendent;
- The Director of Child Nutrition Services;
- 3 Classified employees appointed by their employee organization;
- 3 teachers (elementary, middle, and high school) appointed by their employee organization;
- 1 Principal appointed by their employee organization;
- 5 students (3 middle school and 2 high school) appointed by student government;
- 10 Community/Parent representatives appointed by the Board of Education.

The Wellness Committee shall meet at least six times a year at hours convenient for public participation, and for sufficient time to conduct the group's business.

Index

Recipe Index